PRACTICAL BRONCHOSCOPY

PRACTICAL BRONCHOSCOPY

John Collins MD FRCP
*Consultant Physician, Brompton and
St Stephen's Hospitals, London*

Paul Dhillon MD MRCP
*Consultant Physician, King's Cross and
Ninewells Hospital, Dundee*

Peter Goldstraw MB FRCS
*Consultant Thoracic Surgeon, Brompton, University College
and Middlesex Hospitals, London*

BLACKWELL SCIENTIFIC PUBLICATIONS

OXFORD LONDON EDINBURGH

BOSTON PALO ALTO MELBOURNE

© 1987 by
Blackwell Scientific Publications
Editorial offices:
Osney Mead, Oxford, OX2 0EL
 (*Orders*: Tel. 0865 240201)
8 John Street, London, WC1N 2ES
23 Ainslie Place, Edinburgh, EH3 6AJ
52 Beacon Street, Boston
 Massachusetts 02108, USA
667 Lytton Avenue, Palo Alto
 California 94301, USA
107 Barry Street, Carlton
 Victoria 3053, Australia

First published 1987

Set by Acorn Bookwork, Salisbury
Printed in Great Britain

DISTRIBUTORS

USA
 Year Book Medical Publishers
 35 East Wacker Drive
 Chicago
 Illinois 60601
 (*Orders*: Tel. 312 726–9733)

Canada
 The C.V. Mosby Company
 5240 Finch Avenue East
 Scarborough, Ontario
 (*Orders*: Tel. 416–298–1588)

Australia
 Blackwell Scientific Publications
  (Australia) Pty Ltd
 107 Barry Street
 Carlton, Victoria 3053
 (*Orders*: Tel. (03) 347 0300)

British Library
Cataloguing in Publication Data

Collins, John. *1938—*
 Practical Bronchoscopy
 1. Bronschoscope and bronchoscopy
 I. Title   II. Dhillon, Paul
 III. Goldstraw, Peter
 616.2′307545   RC734.B7
 ISBN 0-632-01367-2

Contents

Not but that many useful things
might be learned by that book,
but he was laughed at
because that art was not to be taught by words,
but practice.

THE COMPLEAT ANGLER
Izaak Walton

Preface

Writing a book describing bronchoscopy involves the application of verbal descriptions to what are essentially nonverbal functions combining delicate proprioceptive and spatial orientation with visual recognition.

The scientific development and initial application of fibreoptic instrumentation was the work of Professor Hopkins at Imperial College London, but most of the subsequent technological developments and refinements have come from the Japanese Optical Industry, and at present the most effective and elegant instruments are all of Japanese manufacture.

The introduction of fibrescopes has revolutionized the investigation of many diseases affecting the airways and has been extended to provide indirect access to the rest of the lungs beyond the airway system. Fibreoptic bronchoscopy is probably the most useful advance in practical investigation of lung disease of the last 25 years. It has made examination of the respiratory tract under local anaesthesia a far less barbaric procedure which the vast majority of patients can readily tolerate with only mild premedication.

Initially it was thought that the very small biopsies produced would present a major disadvantage compared with the larger ones available with the rigid instrument, but pathologists and their staff rapidly accommodated to this problem and the greater range of vision and penetration of the fibrescope compared with the rigid instrument has meant that a high yield of positive biopsies can be obtained.

Making use of the greater flexibility of the fibrescope and the mobility of the tip through an increasingly wide range, albeit in one plane, does not require different skills from those needed with the rigid instrument. For both instruments the operator must develop subtle, proprioceptive and spatial senses transferred from the hand two or three feet to the distal end of the instrument within the patient. Visual orientation within the respiratory tract is probably much easier than in the upper gastrointestinal tract, for the anatomy of the airways, even with its uncommon variations, is much more formalized than that of the oesophagus and stomach. Once the map of the trachea, main lobar and segmental bronchi has been committed to memory, transference to the realities of the inside of the airways is a relatively simple matter. Verbal descriptions of the normal tracheobronchial tree, malignant growths and other variations in pathology are but poor substitutes for the experienced eye and much of the quality of that experience cannot be conveyed in words.

Much effort has been expended in the past trying to prove the superiority of rigid or fibreoptic bronchoscopy for investigating individual problems. This phase is now passed and each technique is recognized to have a part in the investigation of the respiratory system, though specific roles for either instrument may vary with the needs of individual problems. In this book both techniques are covered, not so that the reader may choose one or the other, but rather to be familiar with both.

1 Instruments and layout

TEACHING METHODS

Most of the fibreoptic instruments available and most of the telescopes used with rigid bronchoscopes provide a means by which a second observer may share what the operator sees down the instrument (Fig. 1.1). This observer, however, lacking the simultaneous proprioceptive and spatial orientation of the operator, often finds it difficult to appreciate how the instrument has arrived, where it is and what is visible.

Several models of the airways are available as aids to teaching novice bronchoscopists (Fig. 1.2). These are of limited value, and after 1 or 2 hours have been spent in learning to handle the bronchoscope with the model, the novice should be allowed to gain experience with patients.

It is usual to begin by allowing the learner to handle the bronchoscope after an examination has been completed but before it is removed from the patient. The instructor should then progress as rapidly as possible to introducing the instruments.

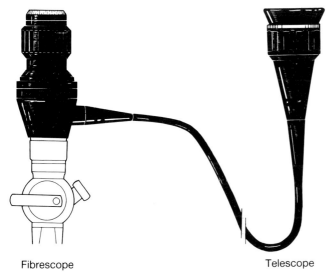

Fibrescope   Telescope

Fig. 1.1 The head of the bronchoscope with the lecturescope or side-viewing attachment in position.

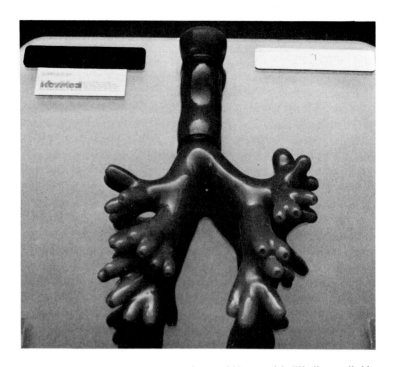

Fig. 1.2 Plastic model of airways used as teaching material. (Kindly supplied by KeyMed, Southend-on-Sea.)

Thereafter the development of the various techniques proceeds at the pace of the individual learner but it is difficult to give figures of the number of bronchoscopies that must be performed before an operator has become competent.

As with all human skills, there is a wide variation in the speed of learning between individuals; and also the range of pathologies available for gaining experience varies from unit to unit. To gain simple proprioceptive, spatial and visual competence with bronchoscopes probably requires a minimum of 3 months, even in busy units, and full competence for the range of procedures that can be performed with modern bronchoscopes needs something nearer 6–12 months and on average more than 100 bronchoscopies.

The spatial arrangement of the airways is easier to appreciate at rigid bronchoscopy. This, and the more limited examination of the bronchial tree possible with this instrument perhaps make it easier to learn to use. As general anaesthesia is usually used for rigid bronchoscopy it provides a useful introduction for the novice before progressing to the fibreoptic instrument. Similarly, when fibrescopy has for any reason to be performed through an endotracheal tube under general anaesthesia, novices can gain helpful experience of spatial orientation and manipulation of the instrument without additional discomfort to the patient.

Photography may be undertaken with the flexible or rigid instrument, but the latter produces better results. Video cameras may be attached to either instrument, producing valuable teaching aids.

FIBREOPTICS

All fibreoptic instruments contain both light-transmitting bundles and separate viewing bundles of glass fibres (Fig. 1.3). Except in the smallest of fibreoptic bronchoscopes there are usually two light-transmitting bundles and one viewing bundle.

Each bundle contains many thousands of fine glass fibres of $10\,\mu$m diameter. Light entering either end of a fibre is transmitted by repeated internal reflections down its length (Fig. 1.4). The enormous advantage of fibreoptics is that the internal reflections continue along the length of the fibre even when it is bent through extreme degrees in its longitudinal axis.

The viewing bundle is the most complicated and expensive part of the instrument. For the image transmitted along a fibreoptic bundle to be useful it must be 'coherent', i.e. the individual components of any image entering the distal end of the viewing bundle must be orientated exactly the same way at the proximal end to enter the observer's eye, so that the image is not inverted or transposed left to right. This 'coherence' is produced by ensuring

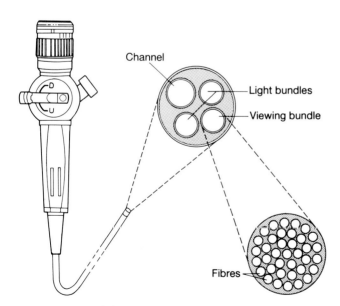

Channel

Light bundles

Viewing bundle

Fibres

Fig. 1.3 Fibreoptic bundles. A magnified image of the distal tip of the bronchoscope showing the two light bundles, the single viewing bundle and the biopsy channel.

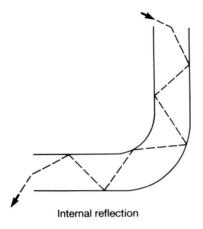

Internal reflection

Fig. 1.4 Light entering either end of the fibre is internally reflected in the bundles and is able to pass round a bend.

that whatever the relative position of each fibre at the distal end of the bundle, this position is maintained at the proximal end. The method of aligning thousands of fibres is the closely guarded secret of successful production of fibrescopes (Fig. 1.5).

Every individual glass fibre has a coating of glass of much lower optical density which prevents light leaking from the interior of the fibre. This coating is not light-transmitting and so produces a dark surrounding to each fibre in the image seen. Fibrescopes with the best optical performances have this interference reduced to a minimum, but inevitably the image does have some element of a grid superimposed upon it and the image quality is unlikely ever to equal that of a rigid lens system.

Current instruments are all made with a distal viewing lens of fixed focal length united to the bundles. At the viewing end of the

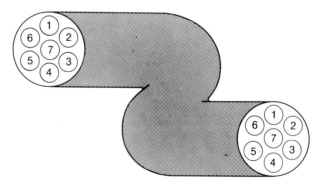

Fig. 1.5 Viewing bundle. Diagrammatic representation of a transmitted image along a fibreoptic bundle. Bundles which begin at the top of the image of the distal end of the fibre must be in the same position at the proximal end for 'Coherence'. e.g. 1.

fibrescope the image is reconstructed and transmitted to the eye with a focusing lens which can be corrected for the refraction differences of the observer's eye.

All modern fibrescopes use cold light from an external high intensity source transmitted down the light-carrying bundles. The fibres of these light bundles do not need to be coherent and can be arranged randomly. Light from the source is conducted to the fibrescope through a connecting cord of such fibres.

THE BRONCHOSCOPY UNIT

Fibreoptic bronchoscopy under local anaesthesia is now a well-established outpatient practice in many hospitals, but the current practice of rigid bronchoscopy using general anaesthesia is mostly performed in conventional operating theatres or recovery rooms. The following details refer to the needs for fibreoptic bronchoscopy (Fig. 1.6).

The demands of space and cost usually dictate that bronchoscopists must use facilities shared with other disciplines especially gastrointestinal endoscopy. The minimal requirements for an effective bronchoscopy service, however, are less than those

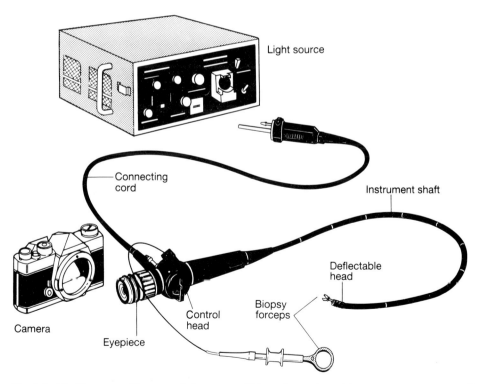

Fig. 1.6   The fibrescope with camera, light source and biopsy forceps in position.

needed for a minor operations theatre or gastrointestinal endoscopy suite where the problems of providing cleanliness and
sterility are greater. Although radiographic screening with a
portable image intensifier is a useful adjunct to some bronchoscopy procedures, it is by no means essential.

A converted kitchen can make an ideal bronchoscopy room and
we have performed many hundreds of bronchoscopies in such a
room measuring $5\,m \times 2.5\,m$ $(13\,m^2)$ (Fig. 1.7). This provides
adequate sink and work surfaces for cleansing apparatus, clean
surfaces for laying out instruments and adequate cupboard space
for the operator at the bedside, for two assistants and an observer
and for access with rarely needed apparatus such as cardiac
defibrillators and ventilators. An oxygen supply and mechanical
suction are essential and overhead lighting which can be dimmed
is useful. Secure storage space for bronchoscopes separate from
this room is advisable.

The amount of sedation usually required and desirable for
patients for fibrescopy is less than that used for gastrointestinal
endoscopy. Many subjects now attend as outpatients and are
given some simple intravenous premedication. Those in hospital
are usually brought in and returned by chair, so a small waiting
area is invaluable. A general air of cheerful informality is helpful
and patients feel more relaxed when the atmosphere does not
resemble that of an operating theatre suite.

The average District General Hospital of 400–500 beds will

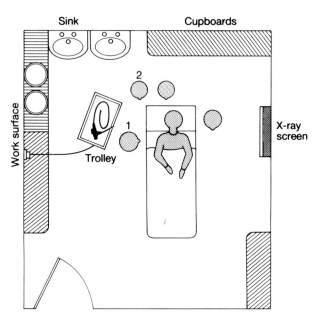

Fig. 1.7 Plan of a suitable bronchoscopy room showing the patient surrounded
by a bronchoscopist (1), nurse (2), and two observers.

generate between three and 10 bronchoscopies a week and these can usually be accommodated in two sessions. Larger institutions performing 750–1000 bronchoscopies per year usually need a larger unit and more sessions.

Most forms of mobile radiological image intensifier increase the space needed for the unit and a room at least 5 m × 7 m is necessary if such equipment is used with bronchoscopy. Wherever possible it is helpful to have the washing up facilities and sterilization equipment in a separate space.

A typical operating theatre table is an unnecessary expense for most units, but if the bronchoscopy couch is adjustable for height this does allow short or tall bronchoscopists greater comfort. Most physicians using fibrescopes prefer the frontal approach, standing on the right side of the couch with the patient semi-recumbent, legs horizontal, with the trunk supported at 45° with the head resting comfortably on a pillow (Fig. 1.8). For this purpose ordinary examination couches of the kind supplied in outpatient departments, are fine. These can be used with a papertowel roll dispenser in place of normal bedding. It is convenient to have the fixtures for the suction trap attached to the couch.

For holding the bronchoscopy light source and bronchoscope, a number of elegant proprietary trolleys are available but are expensive and unnecessary where a unit is established with limited funds (Fig. 1.9). The light source and accessories can be used from a simple kitchen unit cabinet for a fraction of the cost of a special trolley.

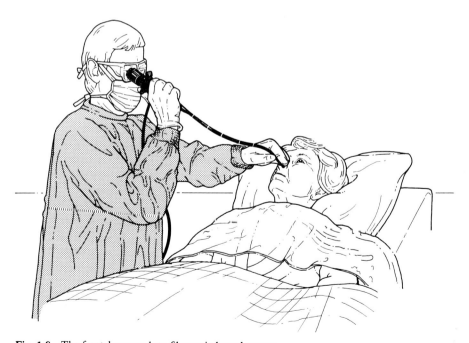

Fig. 1.8 The frontal approach to fibreoptic bronchoscopy.

7

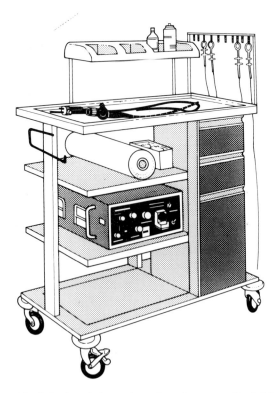

Fig. 1.9 A typical proprietary bronchoscopy trolley holding the light source and other equipment.

2 Anatomy and physiology of the conducting airways

An understanding of the normal anatomy and endoscopic appearance of the airways is essential for the practice of bronchoscopy. Common normal variations must also be appreciated if pathological change is to be recognized. Standard textbooks, cadaveric dissection and various training aids are a helpful introduction but the endoscopic appearance of the moving, breathing and coughing larynx and tracheobronchial tree can only be learned during bronchoscopy.

THE UPPER AIRWAY

The upper airway is held to comprise the nose, pharynx and larynx (Fig. 2.1). Careful fibrescopic examination of these areas is essential to the investigation of haemoptysis, persistent hoarseness and inexplicable cough.

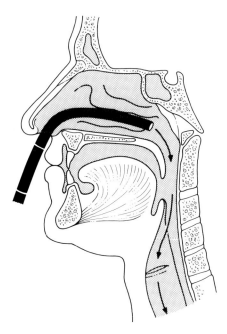

Fig. 2.1 The upper airway. The fibrescope passing beneath the middle turbinate, through the nose to pass back over the soft palate.

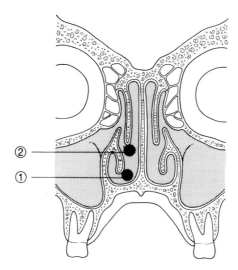

Fig. 2.2 The anterior view of the nasal passages. Two most common sites which will admit the passage of a fibrescope, beneath the inferior turbinate (1), and less commonly, the junction of the middle and inferior turbinates (2).

The majority of bronchoscopic examinations in the Caucasian and Negro races are performed through the nose but in the Japanese, because the nasal passages are generally smaller the fibrescope usually has to be passed through the mouth.

The nasal passages

In the normal adult the nasal airway narrows behind the nostril at the mucocutaneous junction before leading into the inner main nasal passage (Fig. 2.2). The roof of the nasal cavity is formed by the cribriform plate and the palate forms its floor. From the lateral wall project a system of complex folded nasal turbinates which considerably increase the surface area of the mucosa and the resistance to airflow. The medial wall of the nasal cavity is formed by the flat septum.

The superficial and submucosal vascular beds can dilate rapidly in response to irritation, infection and emotion and the thickness of the mucosa of the turbinate may increase up to 4 mm in a few minutes. The relative dilatation of these vascular beds determines the thickness and colour of the nasal mucosa.

The pharynx

Posteriorly, the nasal passages open into the nasopharynx through the choanae and at this point the airway makes an almost 90° turn caudally onto the posterior nasopharyngeal wall. The inferior border of the nasal septum ends and arches to the top of the nasopharynx. The eustachian tubes enter the lateral wall of the nasopharynx at this site and lying between their orifices on the posterior wall are the adenoids.

The calibre and shape of airway in the nasopharynx and oropharynx are determined by contraction of the muscles of the soft palate, tongue, pharynx and larynx as well as the amount of lymphoid tissue in the ring formed by the adenoids, tonsils, base of the tongue and pharynx (Waldeyer's Ring). The oropharynx leads directly to the larynx and here the epiglottis projects upwards onto the base of the tongue, anteriorly.

The larynx

The larynx connects the oropharynx above to the trachea below (Fig. 2.3). It is composed of a system of articulating cartilages of which the most important and strongest is the cricoid, which is the only complete cartilaginous ring in the respiratory tract. The inferior cornuae of the thyroid cartilage are attached to the posterolateral wall of the cricoid cartilage where some degree of rotation and anterior movement of the thyroid cartilage can occur. The epiglottis arises from the posterior aspect of the anterior plate of the thyroid cartilage and sweeps upwards and along the base of the tongue.

The recurrent laryngeal nerve provides the motor innervation to all the intrinsic laryngeal muscles apart from the cricothyroid which is supplied by the superior laryngeal nerve. Injury to the left recurrent laryngeal nerve, a frequent occurrence with mediastinal neoplasms, results in displacement of the affected vocal cord towards the midline because of the unopposed indirect adductor action of the cricothyroid muscle. This adductor effect of the cricothyroid muscles is indirect because it is mediated by rotation of the thyroid cartilage on the cricoid cartilage effectively stretch-

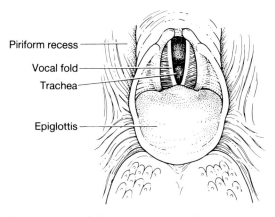

Piriform recess

Vocal fold

Trachea

Epiglottis

Fig. 2.3 A typical view as seen through a fibrescope inserted from the front of the patient.

ing the vocal cord and pulling it to the midline. Much more rarely, injury to the right recurrent laryngeal nerve may occur at the neck or at the thoracic inlet. Mediastinal extension of intrathoracic malignancy, even if right-sided, usually affects the left nerve because of the longer intrathoracic course and proximity of the latter nerve to the mediastinal lymphatic chain.

THE LOWER AIRWAYS

These comprise the trachea, bronchi and bronchioles.

The trachea

The trachea is attached above to the cricoid cartilage by the cricotracheal membrane at the level of the sixth cervical vertebra. It extends through the neck into the upper mediastinum and bifurcates into right and left main bronchi at the level of the sternal angle in front and the fourth thoracic vertebra behind (Fig. 2.4). In the adult the trachea is approximately 12–14 cm in length. Its lower end is attached to the dorsal wall of the pericardial sac and to the diaphragm by the bronchopericardial membrane which is a broad, dense connective tissue structure.

Approximately half the trachea is extrathoracic and the rest is intrathoracic, so that the two halves are subjected to different forces during the respiratory cycle. Both upper and lower ends are attached to mobile structures with the result that the dimensions of the trachea are constantly changing with movements of the head and neck above, and the diaphragm below. The upper part may move as much as 7 cm during extreme flexion–extension movements of the neck and the lower part moves several centimetres during normal respiration and up to 5 cm during coughing or sneezing.

The tracheal wall consists of the larger ventrolateral part containing the cartilages and the flat dorsal muscular wall. The 16–20 tracheal cartilages are incomplete rings, open dorsally, in roughly the shape of a horseshoe, but this is variable and they may be staple or arch-shaped in cross-section.

The cartilages are connected to each other by a fibrous membrane composed of collagen and elastic fibres arranged in a lattice with glandular tissue interspersed between the fibres. The mobile muscular dorsal wall is mainly composed of transverse smooth-muscle fibres connecting the posterior tips of the tracheal cartilages. Collagen and elastic fibres also form a longitudinal band down the length of the trachea along the posterior tips of the cartilages. This adds to the elastic recoil of the dorsal wall of the trachea following deformation. Glandular tissue is also present in this part of the tracheal wall. The mucosa and submucosa of the

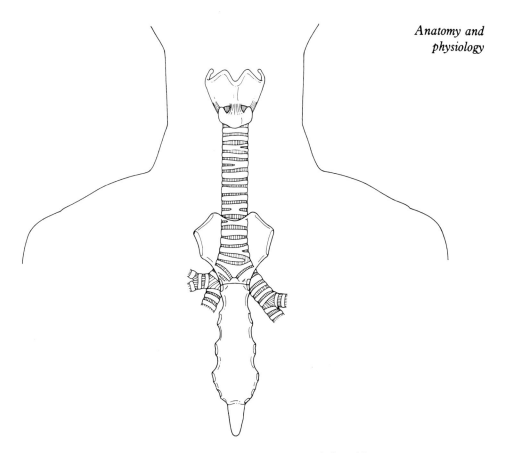

Fig. 2.4   The relationship of the bifurcation of the trachea and main bronchi to the manubrium sterni.

tracheal wall varies in thickness, being thinnest over the cartilages and thickest over the dorsal muscular wall where longitudinal folds may appear as the muscle is contracted. These layers are intimately bound to the cartilaginous rings.

The carina is a concave spur at the distal end of the trachea where it bifurcates into the right and left main bronchi. It is composed of a saddle-shaped carinal cartilage, an interbronchial ligament and the attachment of the fibres of the bronchopericardial membrane. These relatively inflexible structures maintain the sharp angle of the carina.

Viewed endoscopically, the posterior wall of the trachea is relatively flat and protrudes slightly into the tracheal space, especially in expiration. The anterolateral wall forms a rigid arch because of the cartilages. The pressure of the thyroid gland in its upper part may give the trachea an ovoid cross-section at this level. Just above the tracheal bifurcation pulsations can usually be seen where the aortic arch crosses the trachea transversely on its left wall.

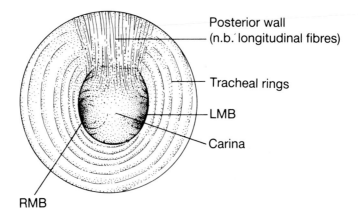

Posterior wall
(n.b. longitudinal fibres)

Tracheal rings

LMB

Carina

RMB

Fig. 2.5 The posterior wall of the trachea, trachea cartilage rings and the carina with right and left main bronchi (RMB = right main bronchus; LMB = left main bronchus).

During inspiration (Fig. 2.5) the trachea dilates to develop an almost circular lumen and in expiration the mobile dorsal wall encroaches into the lumen to produce a kidney-shaped cross-section. These changes in shape are exaggerated during forced inspiration and coughing and are particularly noticeable in children when the trachea may appear flattened ventrodorsally. This change in cross-section of the tracheal lumen serves to amplify the changes in airflow in the trachea during expiration. The most common deformity of the trachea of the cross-section due to intrinsic changes of the normal anatomical structures is the so-called 'scabbard' deformity in which the cross-section is narrowed in the transverse plain (Fig. 2.6).

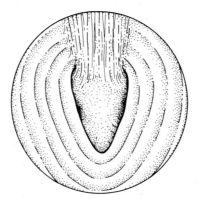

Fig. 2.6 The scabbard type trachea flattened in the transverse plane.

The bronchi

The trachea divides into the right and left main (or primary) bronchi at the carina (Fig. 2.7). The carina is usually vertical in the ventrodorsal plane but may lie at an angle to this plane.

The segment of a lobe ventilated by a segmental bronchus is usually well delineated from neighbouring segments by almost complete planes of connective tissue. This segmental anatomy of the lungs is of considerable importance, as disease may be confined by this to one or two segments of a lobe and may provide useful planes of dissection in surgery. Each segment is named by the position it occupies in a lobe of the lung and the corresponding bronchus carries the same name (Fig. 2.8).

In general most bronchial branches arise from bifurcation of the preceding airway. The resulting branches are smaller than the parent stem bronchus but their combined total cross-sectional area is greater so that the total cross-section of the airways increases rapidly and progressively from trachea to bronchioles.

Bronchial wall structure changes gradually with changes in the size of the airways. The larger bronchi, main stem and lower lobe

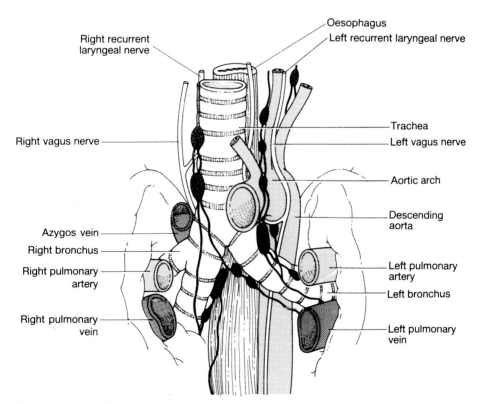

Fig. 2.7 The anterior relations of the trachea and main bronchi to the lungs, main vessels, lymph nodes and nerves.

15

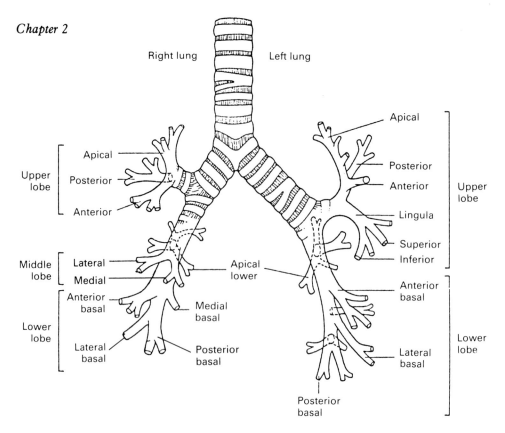

Fig. 2.8 The anterior view of the main bronchi, lobar bronchi and segmental divisions.

bronchi, have cartilages similar to the trachea forming incomplete rings ventrolaterally with membraneous dorsal walls. Medium sized bronchi, upper and middle lobe and segmental bronchi, have large irregular plates of cartilage. In contrast to larger bronchi, these bronchi have complete muscular and elastic layers, the fibres being arranged as an encompassing helix. There is also an increase in mucus-secreting glandular tissue with increase in size of bronchi. The small bronchi, i.e. all those peripheral to segmental bronchi, have small irregular patches of cartilage with few glands. The wall is mainly composed of muscle, collagen and elastic fibres. Plates of cartilage are usually still located at bifurcations of bronchi. In more peripheral regions of the lung the plates of cartilage become more and more isolated and eventually disappear completely at the level of the bronchioles.

In the trachea and large bronchi the muscle layer lies dorsally bridging the gap between the tips of the cartilages. More peripherally as the incomplete rings of cartilage become irregular and patchy, the muscle attachments become progressively more ventral until a complete ring of muscle is formed. At this stage, i.e. segmental bronchi, the bronchial wall consists of loosely organized connective tissue with a rich vascular network between the muscular layer and the bronchial epithelium.

Contraction of the bronchial wall muscle at these sites will result in narrowing of the whole circumference of the airway rather than just the posterior wall as in the trachea and larger bronchi. The mucosal and submucosal layers can collapse readily into the lumen as they are not adherent to any cartilage. Excessive suction pressure applied via a bronchoscope may cause such collapse of the airway and damage the mucosal and submucosal layers as they are sucked into the aspiration channel. If there is bronchial wall thickening and mucosal oedema as in chronic bronchitis the damage will be greater.

Through their attachments to the trachea proximally and lung parenchyma distally, bronchi lengthen and widen with inspiration and shorten and narrow with expiration. The elastic fibres in the bronchial wall are arranged circumferentially and longitudinally providing the elastic recoil promoting decrease of lung volume. The bronchial musculature is arranged in a helical manner and this provides a mechanism for active alterations in both calibre and length of the airways. Contraction of this geodesic helix of muscle makes the bronchial wall more rigid, resisting collapse.

Endoscopically the normal bronchial mucosa appears as a glossy pink membrane. Small vessels may be seen around the carina and in the walls of the main bronchi. These are branches of the bronchial circulation which is systemic in origin and supplies the structures of the intrathoracic airways. The gloss is due to the presence of the normal surface layer of mucus. Small collections of mucus are commonly encountered in normal airways, but if repeated aspiration is required to keep the field of vision clear then excess secretions are probably present. With increasing age a gradual atrophy of the submucosa occurs, the mucosa appears paler and the cartilages and carinae become thinner and sharper.

The normal delicate mucosa is easily injured even by rubbing with the tip of the bronchoscope or by injudicious suction. A reactive hyperaemia follows and this may progress to bruising or even bleeding.

Branching of the bronchial tree

The main branches of the bronchial tree out to the segmental bronchi may be inspected but not necessarily entered with the rigid bronchoscope. One advantage of the fibrescope is that more peripheral airways become visible out to subsegmental levels. A knowledge of the variations of the normal anatomy of these peripheral airways thus becomes important. Some degree of normal variation of the branching of the bronchial tree occurs;

17

this is rare at the lobar level, but not uncommon at the segmental level and commonplace with the more peripheral branches.

The usual lobar branches of the right main bronchus are the upper, middle and lower lobe bronchi and that of the left main bronchus are the upper and lower lobe bronchi. Rare variations of this branching which may occur are:

1 abnormalities in the direction that bronchi branch from the stem bronchi

2 absence of portions of bronchi and associated lack of the middle lobe

3 formation of a part of the upper lobe as a result of branching off of a bronchus from the right main bronchus (accessory bronchus)

4 cystic or diverticular formation of an abnormally small lobe which is not present in the 'normal' lung

5 subdivision of the right upper lobe due to accessory or aberrant bronchi branching out just above the tracheal carina

Variations of bronchial branching are commoner in the right lung. Very rarely mirror-image anatomy may present in *situs inversus*.

Each lobar bronchus branches into two to six segmental bronchi.

The clinical nomenclature of the segmental bronchi has been adapted from Jackson & Huber (1943) with the addition of the subapical or subsuperior lower lobe branch. Because of the considerable variation in branching which occurs at a segmental level these are described here.

RIGHT LUNG

The right main bronchus is usually the larger of the two and deviates less from the tracheal axis than does the left, as the latter crosses beneath the aortic arch and other mediastinal structures. Any foreign body entering the trachea under the influence of gravity will usually fall into the right bronchial tree. This applies to inhaled foreign bodies and any instrument or endotracheal tube inserted by an unskilled operator.

The right main bronchus divides into three lobar branches, the upper, middle and lower lobes and the left divides into two, the upper and lower lobes.

The lobar or secondary bronchi, in turn divide into segmental or tertiary bronchi, which supply discrete segments of lung.

The right intermediate bronchus is of importance to the surgeon since it separates the origin of the middle and lower lobe bronchi from that of the upper lobe bronchus. Hence tumours approaching the origin of middle or lower lobe bronchi may possibly be resected preserving the upper lobe if the intermediate

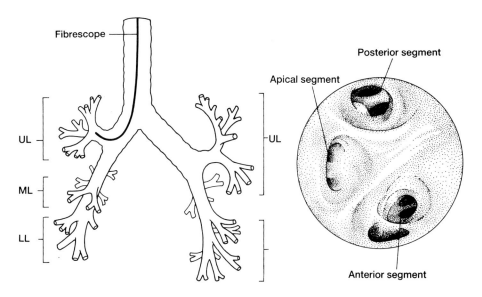

Fig. 2.9 Normal view of the right upper lobe (UL = upper lobe; ML = middle lobe; LL = lower lobe)

bronchus is uninvaded. Similarly upper lobe tumours encroaching on the descending bronchus may be resected with a sleeve of descending bronchus, allowing preservation of the lower and middle lobes.

The right upper lobe bronchus divides into three segmental bronchi, the apical, posterior and anterior which supply segments of the same name (Fig. 2.9). Six different types of variation of branching have been described (Nagaishi 1972).

Type I
the most common occurring in 40% of cases; all three segmental bronchi branch out independently of each other.

Type II
occurring in 24% of cases; the posterior segmental bronchus branches independently and the other two form a common trunk.

Type III
occurring in 14% of cases; the anterior branch is independent and the apical and posterior are combined.

Type IV
occurring in 10% of cases; the apical branch is independent and the other two form a common trunk.

Type V
occurring in 10% of cases; the posterior segmental bronchus is absent and all branches arise from the apical and anterior bronchi.

Type VI
occurring in 2% of cases; the apical bronchus is absent and branches arise from the other two segmental bronchi.

19

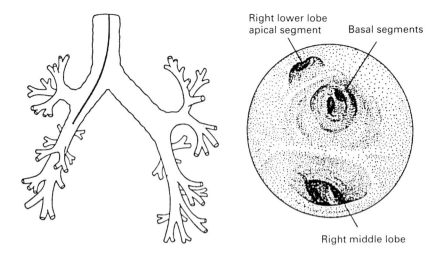

Fig. 2.10 Normal view of the right middle lobe.

The right middle lobe bronchus divides into two segmental bronchi, the lateral and the medial. In approximately 70% of cases each arises independently and the two are of the same calibre. In 18–22%, the medial branch is smaller and branches off the lateral bronchus (Fig. 2.10). Less often (6–18%) the lateral bronchus is smaller and appears to arise from the medial bronchus.

The right lower lobe bronchus usually divides into five segmental bronchi: the apical (or superior) and the four basal bronchi (medical anterior, lateral and posterior) (Fig. 2.11). An additional

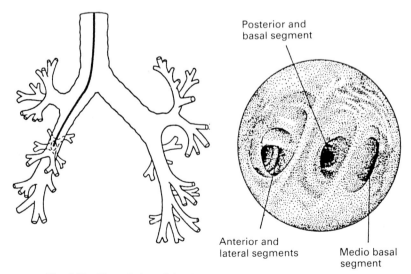

Fig. 2.11 Normal view of the right lower lobe.

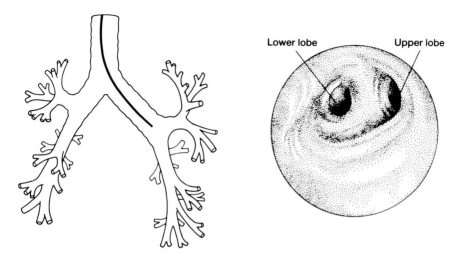

Fig. 2.12 Normal view of the left main bronchus.

subapical (or subsuperior) is also found in 44–60% of cases, usually when the apical, lateral or posterior basal segments are poorly developed. The apical segment usually arises from the posteromedial aspect of the right lower lobe bronchus near its origin and may arise proximal to the middle lobe bronchus. Very rarely it may stem from the posterior wall of the middle lobe bronchus itself. The apical segmental bronchus divides immediately into three (more rarely two) subsegmental bronchi.

Of the other segmental bronchi of the right lower lobe the mediobasal bronchus is always present in the right lung and usually divides into two subsegmental bronchi (Fig. 2.12). It arises proximal to the remaining three basal segmental bronchi, the anterior, lateral and posterior, which diverge out towards the diaphragm. In both right and left lungs, the most common variations of branching of these three basal segmental bronchi is one in which the anterior segmental bronchus arises most proximally from the lower lobe main stem bronchus, and then distally this main stem lobar bronchus divides into the lateral and posterior segmental branches. The second most common variation of branching is where all three segmental bronchi arise independently at the same level. The third common type is that in which the anterior and lateral segmental bronchi arise together proximally and the posterior segmental bronchus forms a separate terminal trunk.

LEFT LUNG

The left main bronchus divides into the left upper and lower bronchi (Fig. 2.12). The left upper lobe bronchus divides into

21

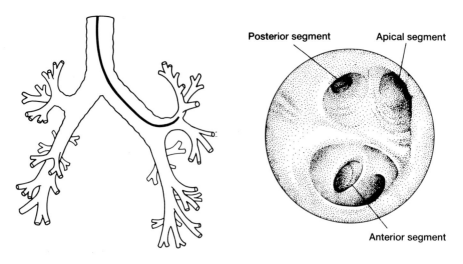

Fig. 2.13 View of the left upper division of the left upper lobe.

two main divisions, the upper and the lingula which correspond to the right upper and middle lobes (Figs 2.13, 2.14). The upper division bronchus usually divides into an apico-posterior and anterior bronchi. The apico-posterior bronchus subsequently forms three segmental bronchi, the first supplying the apex, the second the posterosuperior and posteroinferior regions of the apex and the third the posterolateral region of the lobe. The variations in branching of these segmental bronchi are of three main types:

1 in 62%, the posterolateral segmental bronchus branches off most proximally with the other two segments forming a common trunk

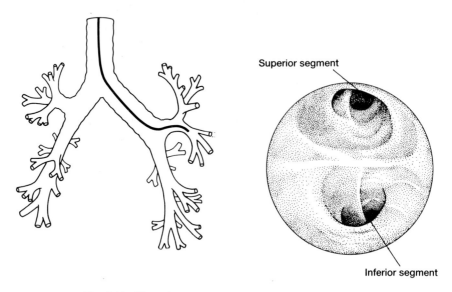

Fig. 2.14 View of the lingula division of the left upper lobe.

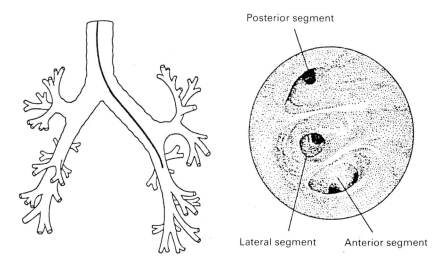

Fig. 2.15 View of the basal segments of the left lower lobe.

2 in 24%, a common trunk is formed by the posterosuperior and posteroinferior bronchi and the posterolateral branches proximally leaving the terminal bronchus to supply the apex of the lobe

3 in 14%, the posterolateral segmental bronchus branches from the anterior rather than the apico-posterior bronchus

The lingula division bronchus of the left upper lobe divides into two segmental bronchi, the superior and inferior branches (Fig. 2.14). Each of these subsequently divides into two subsegmental bronchi.

The left lower lobe bronchial branches are 'mirror-images' of those described for the right except for the absence of the mediobasal segment due to the presence of the heart (Fig. 2.15). Thus the apical or superior segmental bronchus branches most proximally from the posterior wall of the left lower lobe bronchus, followed by the anterior, lateral and posterior segmental bronchi in sequence. Often a subapical (or subsuperior) segmental bronchus is also present distal to the origin of the apical bronchus.

REFLEXES FROM THE CONDUCTING AIRWAYS

In order to appreciate and prevent some of the side-effects and complications which may arise from bronchoscopy, the normal reflex effects of irritation and trauma of the upper and lower airways must be understood. Some of these reflexes, e.g. the cough, cannot be abolished completely and are mainly of nuisance value, but others such as cardiac dysrhythmias, may have more serious consequences.

Upper respiratory tract reflexes

Sneezing is the most obvious respiratory reflex of the nose but causes few problems during transnasal fibrescopy and is usually readily blocked by local anaesthesia. However, the other reflex functions may be active but are less obvious. In conscious man nasal inhalation or irritants may cause rapid, shallow or slow, deep breathing, bronchospasm and variable blood pressure changes.

Touching the nasal mucosa causes an unpleasant sensation and cold saline or water in the nose can cause apnoea and hypertension. Cold air in the nose may also cause bronchoconstriction in asthmatic individuals. The normal relevance of these reflexes is not clear. Apnoea and bronchoconstriction may prevent the inhalation of noxious irritants as may rapid, shallow respirations. The purpose of these reflex effects on the cardiovascular system are even more difficult to understand.

The larynx has similar reflex responses to various stimuli. Epithelial, joint and muscle receptors in the epiglottis as well as of the larynx may be involved. Mechanical stimulation by food or endoscopy can result in coughing, laryngospasm, bronchoconstriction and cardiac dysrhythmias. Similar reflexes can occur following chemical irritation and the larynx probably has the lowest threshold for stimulation of the cough reflex of any part of the conducting airways. If efferent nerve fibres to the larynx are stimulated, coughing results. This in turn causes mucous membrane deformation which suggests the existence of a self-perpetuating reflex arc.

Lower respiratory tract reflexes

Coughing is the main respiratory reflex response to irritation of the lower respiratory tract. The cough reflex consists of a sequence of a deep inspiration, closure of the glottis followed rapidly by a strong expiratory effort and sudden opening of the glottis producing a forceful explosive expiration.

Different regions of the airway vary in their sensitivity to several types of irritant stimuli. In addition to the larynx, the carina and the branching points of the lobar bronchi are the most sensitive to mechanical stimuli. Bronchi beyond the segmental level are relatively insensitive. Conversely, chemical stimuli to cough appear to be more effective in the peripheral airways than in the trachea or large bronchi. The nature of the cough reflex also differs with the two types of stimuli. Chemical stimuli cause a cough preceded by an initial inspiration, while mechanical irritation causes an immediate expiratory effort.

The receptors for the cough reflex consist of fine terminal filaments of nerve fibres which lie between epithelial cells in the superficial ciliary layer. These afferent end-organs are found concentrated in the dorsal, fibromuscular wall of the trachea, the main carina and the junctions between lobar bronchi.

Electrophysiological studies of the vagi in animals suggest that there are probably two types of receptors responding mainly to either mechanical or chemical irritants, with some functional overlap between the two. Receptors responding primarily to mechanical deformation are concentrated in the trachea and carina. Those responding primarily to chemical irritants are found mainly in more peripheral subsegmental bronchi.

The intrathoracic forces that occur during the cough reflex have effects on other systems. Intrathoracic pressure can rise briefly up to 300 mmHg and systemic arterial blood pressure may vary from 50–300 mmHg. Venous and cerebrospinal fluid pressures may reach as high as 300 mmHg and right ventricular pressure may rise by 10 cm H_2O for 30–60 seconds after coughing.

Reflex bronchoconstriction due to constriction of bronchial wall muscle may occur in response to irritant stimuli. This may be a problem with asthmatic patients who have hypersensitive airways which constrict in response to even mild stimuli.

REFERENCES AND FURTHER READING

FENN W. O. & RAHN H., eds (1964) *Handbook of Physiology, Section 3: Respiration*, Vol. 1. American Physiological Society, Washington DC.

JACKSON C. L. & HUBER J. F. (1943) Correlated applied anatomy of the bronchial tree with system of nomenclature. *Dis. Chest* **9**, 319.

NAGAISHI C. (1972) *Functional Anatomy and Histology of the Lung*. University Park Press, Baltimore.

SHIOZAWA M. (1954/5) *Segmental Resection of the Lung* (in Japanese), Vols 1 and 2. Bunkodo, Tokyo.

STRADLING P. (1981) *Diagnostic Bronchoscopy*. Churchill Livingstone, Edinburgh.

3 The procedure of bronchoscopy

BRONCHOSCOPY PROCEDURE

The patient's acceptance of bronchoscopy will be helped by prior adequate explanation and ideally the bronchoscopist should be involved at the stage of initial planning. The bronchoscopist must always assure himself that:

1 the indications for bronchoscopy are adequate
2 risk factors involved are acceptable
3 the patient understands the investigation and has given written consent
4 the patient is fit for general anaesthesia (where appropriate)

Risk factors

There are no absolute contraindications to bronchoscopy provided that the clinical needs merit the risks of the investigation. Major risk factors include bleeding diatheses, irreversible hypoxaemia where the aterial oxygen tension is less than 8 kPa (60 mmHg), serious cardiac dysrhythmias and recent myocardial infarction. Major neck deformities make rigid bronchoscopy difficult or impossible but fibrescopy can still be performed even with atlanto-axial subluxation. Superior vena caval obstruction greatly increases the risk of laryngeal oedema following bronchoscopy. Fibrescopy, however, is much safer than rigid bronchoscopy as the patient can be kept in the sitting position throughout the procedure. Other risk factors include severe airways obstruction, especially with asthma, and severe haemorrhage following biopsy, a particular risk with chronic renal failure; vascular tumours and clotting abnormalities. Rupture of a lung abscess can cause flooding of the airways with pus and widespread aspiration. Lung infection following bronchoscopy is a rare problem in immunocompromised patients.

Infection

Ideally, patients with pulmonary tuberculosis should have had at least 2 weeks effective chemotherapy before bronchoscopy. Where bronchoscopy has been used to establish the diagnosis of tuberculosis the instrument should be sterilized by prolonged immersion in glutaraldehyde or with ethylene oxide. Viral hepatitis and human immunodeficiency virus (HIV) infection are two particular hazards for endoscopists. Present practice is to screen all patients for hepatitis–associated antigen before bronchoscopy and to use a special reserved fibrescope paying particular attention to aseptic techniques using theatre gowns, masks and surgical gloves. All equipment is carefully swabbed with glutaraldehyde after bronchoscopy. The use of goggles or protective spectacles is advised particularly during rigid bronchoscopy where air expired up the bronchoscope may carry contaminated blood or mucus into the endoscopist's eye (*see* Chapter 9).

Informed consent

To allay the patient's understandable anxiety, a full reassuring explanation is helpful. A detailed explanation of the distasteful nature of the local anaesthetic used for the nose and pharynx, and a calm and reassuring bronchoscopist help to augment the effects of premedication. Written consent should be obtained.

Preparation and premedication

The patient should fast completely for 4 hours before bronchoscopy. For emergency examination however, metoclopramide 10 mg i.v. may be advisable. Most experienced bronchoscopists find the amount of premedication needed lessens as their experience increases, and a calm atmosphere with the presence of as few people in the unit as possible, are helpful. Physical contact with the patient by initial handshaking, feeling the pulse or a hand on the shoulder enhances communication and relaxation. Quiet reassurance to the patient aimed at relaxation of muscle tension in the shoulders and arms and encouragement of quiet regular breathing will help in the induction of bronchoscopy.

For fibrescopy the frontal approach allows the operator to make direct visual contact with the patient. The patient should be advised to keep his eyes open throughout the procedure (Fig. 3.1). This improves his tolerance, probably through competitive inhibition of discomfort from the respiratory tract through sensory inhibition produced by simultaneous visual stimuli.

There are many variations in the drugs used for premedication in fibrescopy. One of the commonest is the use of papaveratum (Omnopon) IM, 60 minutes before fibrescopy. The dose is adjusted according to the age, weight and general fitness of the patient. If necessary excessive sedation and hypoventilation can be reversed with the use of a specific antagonist naloxone (Narcan) 0.2–0.4 mg i.v. The half-life of this drug is less than that of the opiates and repeated doses may be necessary. For patients with asthma pethidine 50–100 mg IM is preferable to papavertum

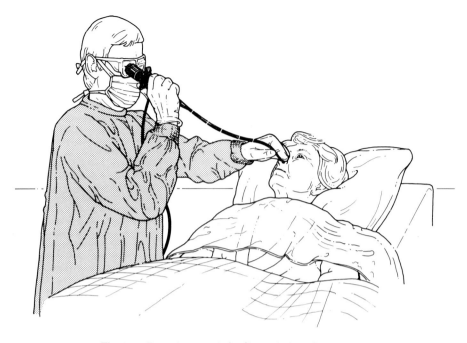

Fig. 3.1 Frontal approach for fibreoptic bronchoscopy.

as it causes less bronchoconstriction. Intravenous diazepam as a lipid emulsion (Diazemuls) is very effective as rapid premedication or to augment sedation during bronchoscopy.

The use of atropine 0.5–1.0 mg IM to reduce salivation, bronchial secretions and the vaso-vagal reflex is probably unnecessary. Where patients with asthma are bronchoscoped, prior inhalation of nebulized salbutamol or terbutaline 30 minutes beforehand helps to prevent or minimize airway obstruction.

TOPICAL ANALGESIA

For children and about 0.1% of adults general anaesthesia is needed for fibrescopy. However the vast majority of procedures are carried out with topical analgesia alone.

The most widely used analgesic is lignocaine (Xylocaine). For bronchoscopy, lignocaine solutions ranging from 1–10% are used and the topical analgesia induced lasts up to 20 minutes. Except for patients with recognized cardiac dysrhythmias, the drug is safe up to a total of about 400 mg. Lignocaine has useful vasoconstrictor properties through inhibition of re-uptake of noradrenaline at sympathetic nerve endings. This shrinks the nasal and pharyngeal mucosa easing the passage of the fibrescope.

Although cocaine is reputedly the best local analgesic with a longer duration of action, of up to an hour, it has a smaller safety margin than lignocaine and presents additional security problems because it is a highly addictive narcotic. Although popular in the United States it has not been widely used in Britain. Tetracaine, which is extremely rapid in onset, has a very narrow therapeutic range and several deaths have been reported with its use.

Serum levels of lignocaine during bronchoscopy vary widely but toxic actions are rarely encountered, and usually occur when the serum level exceeds $6 \mu g/ml$. Such toxic reactions are more likely in the elderly and in the presence of cardiac, renal and hepatic disease. Early signs of toxicity include tremulousness, shivering, talkativeness, dizziness and sedation. More severe reactions including convulsions, unconsciousness, respiratory arrest and cardiovascular collapse can ensue rapidly. Fortunately, such toxic reactions are rare. It is essential that full resuscitation apparatus and medications are always to hand.

Five main techniques for topical analgesia for fibrescopy are available: 'spray as you go', gargling with lignocaine solution, dropper instillation, transtracheal injection and local nerve block.

'Spray as you go'

The 'spray as you go' method is the most widely used and is the instillation of local analgesia through the advancing fibrescope. It is efficient and effective for the larynx, vocal cords and trachea which can be clearly visualized as the fibrescope is advanced and the anaesthetic agent can be applied directly to the next segment to be entered. Aliquots of 0.5–1 ml solution are instilled through the channel of the fibrescope. This allows the amount of analgesia to be kept to a minimum and matched against the effectiveness of the suppression of the cough reflex.

Analgesia for the nose and oropharynx is instituted by the use of lignocaine aerosol. This usually requires 30–50 mg in total. A proprietary 10% lignocaine spray which delivers a metered 10 mg puff per dose is very useful for analgesia in the nose. The first 10 cm of the fibrescope from its distal tip are lubricated using 2% lignocaine gel and once the instrument has been successfully inserted through nose or mouth 4% lignocaine in one or two aliquots of 2 ml (80–160 mg) is instilled under bronchoscopic vision onto the vocal cords and upper airways. This is rapidly effective and once swallowing movements and coughing have ceased the fibrescope can be advanced between the vocal cords. Thereafter 2% lignocaine solution is instilled in aliquots of 2 ml (40 mg) where needed up to a total dose of about 400 mg.

Dropper instillation

This traditional technique is performed with the patient seated erect (indirect laryngeal vision used). The mouth and pharynx are sprayed with 1–2% lignocaine. A malleable curved adapter is attached to a syringe and used to instill 0.5–1 ml aliquots of lignocaine to the base of the tongue, the valleculae (to block superior laryngeal nerve endings), the epiglottis, the adducted vocal cords and the trachea. This is a cumbersome and outdated procedure.

Gargling

Effective analgesia of the glottis and upper airways can be achieved by gargling with mucinous solutions of lignocaine before bronchoscopy. This method however is a little tedious for both patient and bronchoscopist.

Transtracheal instillation

This is performed by injecting local analgesic through the cricothyroid membrane. Transient vigorous coughing is followed by effective analgesia. This seems a rather invasive procedure and it is more difficult to match the dose of analgesic to needs so that the risk of high serum levels with toxic reactions is greater.

Local nerve block

The 'local nerve block' method involves pharyngeal submucosal injections to block the glossopharyngeal nerves and external neck injections to block the superior laryngeal nerves. This 'barbaric' procedure has rarely been used in Britain.

GENERAL ANAESTHESIA

Rigid bronchoscopy

The main difficulty in general anaesthesia for rigid bronchoscopy is to maintain a sealed airway for assisted ventilation. This problem has been circumvented in various ways in the past by using spontaneous respiration, cuirasse ventilation, passing an endotracheal tube alongside the bronchoscope and by pre-oxygenation of the patient. Spontaneous respiration is still popular for paediatric bronchoscopy but the other techniques have all proved inadequate for adults.

Pre-oxygenation for several minutes allows bronchoscopy during apnoea but there is a progressive rise in arterial carbon dioxide tension and the examination cannot safely proceed beyond 3–4 minutes. Interruption, at least temporarily, is necessary to allow ventilation via a face mask or endotracheal tube.

Modern rigid bronchoscopes may be fitted with a proximal eye glass and ventilating side-arm to allow ventilation during the examination. In the adult the bronchoscope does not fit perfectly into the trachea and even with high gas flows, effective ventilation is not achieved. Because the eye glass must be removed to introduce suction, telescopes or biopsy forceps, ventilation is then further reduced. In children such a system may prove the safest available since the bronchoscope is proportionately wider giving a tighter tracheal fit allowing good ventilation but making the use of the Venturi system more hazardous (see below).

Since its introduction in 1967 the Sanders Venturi System has become the most widely used system for ventilation during rigid bronchoscopy in adults. With this technique the patient is kept anaesthetized and paralysed using intravenous agents. Ventilation is achieved by a jet of oxygen through a fine bore needle fixed to the proximal end of the bronchoscope. Air is entrained through and around the bronchoscope to provide a variable oxygen concentration in the gases reaching the distal airways. Expired gases escape around the bronchoscope. The inspired oxygen concentration will vary with the calibre of the needle, the driving pressure of the oxygen and the fit of the bronchoscope within the airways. These factors also affect the pressure generated in the lungs and care must be taken to ensure that the pressure of the oxygen supply from the pipeline or cylinder is not excessive and that the needle is of the correct calibre. For adults a size 16 SWG needle is adequate and oxygen pressure is restricted to 410 kPa. If there is doubt, the system should be checked by immersing the bronchoscope in a cylinder of water and observing the depth of immersion at which air escapes from the end of the bronchoscope. For

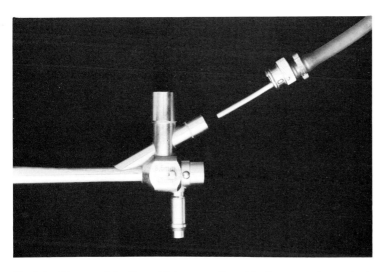

Fig. 3.2 Close-up of the Venturi injector needle and its fitment on the proximal end of the bronchoscope.

children a smaller gauge needle is necessary to avoid generating excessive pressure within the airways.

The bronchoscope must not be wedged within a distal bronchus since excessive pressure may cause air embolization and death. The reader is recommended to study the details of this technique in standard textbooks of anaesthesia (e.g. Gothard & Braithwaite). Using this technique prolonged, safe ventilation is possible permitting unhurried careful examination even in the trying circumstances surrounding removal of a foreign body.

Flexible fibrescopy

As for rigid bronchoscopy, the main problem during fibrescopy under general anaesthesia is the maintenance of adequate ventilation. The most common technique consists of insertion of the fibrescope via an endotracheal tube through which the oxygen and anaesthetic gases are being delivered to the patient (Fig. 3.3). The fibrescope markedly increases resistance to the flow of respiratory

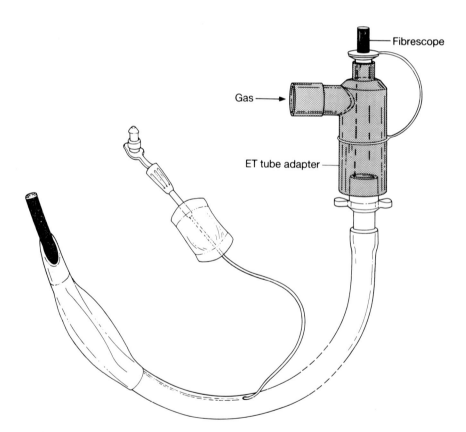

Fibrescope

Gas

ET tube adapter

Fig. 3.3 Fibrescope inserted through an airtight seal in an endotracheal tube for the ventilated patient.

gases, e.g. when a 5 mm fibrescope is used through an 8 mm endotracheal tube, the resistance to flow of gas is increased sufficiently to cause hypercapnia and hypoxia.

To try to minimize this problem anaesthetists use the largest possible endotracheal tube or a specially designed tube for fibrescopy (Medical Engineering, Racine, Wisconsin). This endotracheal tube has a wide upper section (11 m internal diameter) and a narrow lower section that goes through the vocal cords. An 8 mm version of this tube, with a fibrescope in place has a lower resistance to the flow of gases than a 9.5 mm standard endotracheal tube.

A tight seal must be maintained around the fibrescope, at the point where it enters the endotracheal tube, otherwise positive pressure ventilation cannot be maintained. An adaptor which has a diaphragm with a hole in it has been produced. This can be plugged for routine ventilation. With the plug removed the fibrescope can be inserted through the hole in the diaphragm. The seal with the fibrescope is adequate during positive pressure ventilation to prevent leakage of inspired gases.

RIGID BRONCHOSCOPY TECHNIQUE

Following induction of anaesthesia the patient's head is supported on a single pillow so that the head is extended on the neck and the neck is flexed on the shoulders—the so-called 'sniffing rose' position. The head is held extended by the fingers of the endoscopist's left hand, exerting pressure on the upper alveolus and jaw. The bronchoscope in the endoscopist's right hand is then inserted behind the tongue and gently levered forward to view the epiglottis which is lifted forwards to show the larynx. The bronchoscope should never be pressed against the upper teeth or alveolus as it should always be in contact with the dorsum of the endoscopist's left fingers (Fig. 3.4).

The larynx is gently intubated by insinuating the instrument between the vocal cords. Throughout the rest of the examination the instrument is kept away from the upper teeth or alveolus by the thumb of the bronchoscopist's left hand pushing upwards on the instrument and by the fingers of the left hand protecting the teeth. Ventilation is continued by the anaesthetist using the methods discussed above, monitoring the patient's chest wall movement, skin colour, heart rate and peripheral pulse. A thorough bronchoscopic examination should include inspection of the larynx, trachea, carina and all segmental bronchi on both sides. It is customary to examine the normal side first so that any bleeding produced by biopsy in the abnormal side does not obscure examination of the normal side. Right angle telescopes should be used to inspect the upper lobes and may also give a

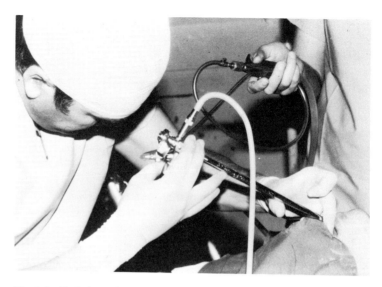

Fig. 3.4 Technique of insertion of rigid bronchoscope, emphasising the protection of the upper teeth and alveolus by the operator's left hand. The Saunder's injection device can be seen in the anaesthetist's right hand.

better view into the apical segment of each lower lobe. The forward viewing telescopes will extend vision beyond the reach of the bronchoscope into the segments of the middle and lower lobes. If any bleeding is produced by biopsy it should be completely controlled before removing the instrument. This can usually be achieved with gentle suction a few millimetres from the bleeding point. This aspect should not be hurried and may require some extension of the anaesthetic time.

Once bleeding has ceased and the examination is completed the bronchoscope is withdrawn and ventilation with the face mask reinstituted until spontaneous ventilation returns and is found to be adequate. The patient is then turned onto the abnormal side to recover completely. By keeping the abnormal side dependent, soiling of the unaffected side by blood or sputum is thus prevented.

FIBRESCOPY TECHNIQUE

Insertion of the fibrescope through the nose requires minimal co-operation of the patient and little risk of damage to the instrument. If the instrument has to go through the mouth it is advisable to use a guard tube in the conscious patient to prevent damage of the instrument from the patient's teeth (Fig. 3.5). The fibrescope can also be introduced through the rigid bronchoscope. The most common source of pain from the fibrebronchoscope is

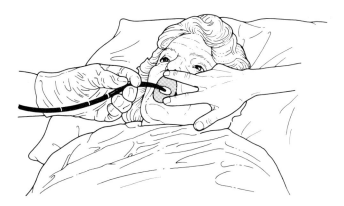

Fig. 3.5 Fibrescope being passed through a guard for introduction through the mouth with an assistant holding the guard in place with two fingers.

deformation of the intra-nasal mucosa. This can be minimized by preventing undue sideways movement of the shaft of the bronchoscope if the operator holds it between the index finger and thumb, close to the patient's nostril (Fig. 3.6). It is advisable to have expertise in all methods but over 90% of bronchoscopies can be performed through the nose.

Nasal insertion of the fibrescope is the most comfortable for the patient as it does not interfere with swallowing and there is less tendency to gag and vomit. It has the immense advantage that the fibrescope cannot be bitten by the patient. However, unless the operator is experienced and careful, nasal insertion can be painful as the turbinates and mucosal lining are sensitive. This can be minimized if lateral movements of the fibrescope tip in the

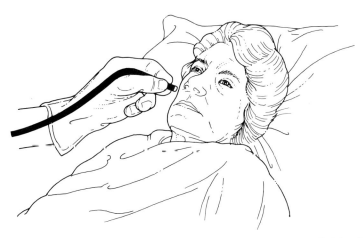

Figer 3.6 The distal end of the bronchoscope is carefully controlled by the bronchoscopist's left hand to prevent damage and distortion of delicate nasal tissue and associated pain.

nose are minimized by keeping the fibrescope controlled by the left-hand (i.e. the hand not used for the fibrescope control mechanism in a right-handed bronchoscopist) (*see* Fig. 3.6).

Insertion through the mouth is used where the nasal passages are too small and it is essential to use a mouth guard to prevent injury to the fibrescope. Passing the fibrescope through an endotracheal tube is simple but in the conscious patient it is an uncomfortable procedure. It has been recommended as an essential technique to control haemorrhage and to avoid the effects of widespread intrapulmonary sepsis. This is questionable.

In practice it has proved easy to use the fibrescope as an introducer for an endotracheal tube where profuse haemorrhage is occurring during bronchoscopy. The endotracheal tube with a minimum internal diameter of 8.5 mm is first advanced up the shaft of the fibrescope which has been removed. The fibrescope is then re-inserted into the larynx and the vocal cords are visualized as the fibrescope is passed into the trachea. More lubricant is then applied to the outside of the endotracheal tube and it is passed over the bronchoscope into place in the trachea.

The position of the patient during bronchofibrescopy depends on the personal preference of the bronchoscopist and comfort of

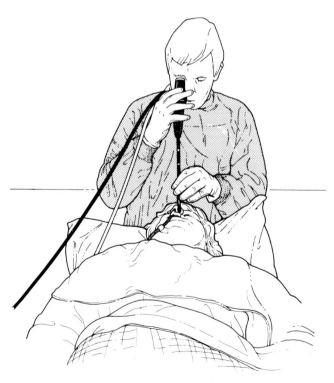

Fig. 3.7 Fibreoptic bronchoscopy from the alternate position, behind the patient.

the patient. Some bronchoscopists prefer to face the sitting or lying patient whilst others stand behind the head of the lying patient (Fig. 3.7). Face to face contact with the frontal approach generally proves valuable to maintain rapport between patient and bronchoscopist. An advantage of standing behind the head of the supine patient is that the spatial orientation of the bronchial tree is then the same for both flexible and rigid bronchoscopes, which may be of importance for bronchoscopists who practise both methods but have difficulty in transposing images.

Fibrescopy procedure

The patient is seated comfortably with legs horizontal and trunk and head supported at 30–45° with a pillow under the head. The bronchoscopist stands to the right of the couch and the assistant behind the patient's head.

Lignocaine solution (4 or 10%) is sprayed from an atomizer into each nostril, the fauces and posterior pharyngeal wall, the patient having been first warned that the initial effects are an unpleasant stinging and taste. Within 2–3 minutes the fibrescope lubricated with lignocaine gel can be introduced into the nose or mouth. Once the bronchoscope has passed through the nose or mouth, supplemental oxygen can be given through a nasal cannula into the unoccupied nostril.

The bronchoscopist should wear a clean gown and disposable gloves. If the gloves have been dusted with powder this must first be washed off to prevent starch granules contaminating the trap specimen and causing confusion in interpretation of the specimens at microscopy.

The fibrescope should be inspected and if necessary the lens cleaned with sterile gauze moistened with sterile saline. The flexible fibrescope is a delicate and expensive apparatus. It must at all times be handled with care to avoid damage to the fibres. Knocking the shaft or tip against furniture and bending or kinking the shaft or tip with undue force must be avoided. The central channel and the polythene connecting tube should be flushed by aspirating sterile saline. To reduce fogging the distal lens can be wiped with silicone or soapy water. The fibrescope shaft should be lubricated with sterile 2% lignocaine jelly and some of this jelly can also be applied into the nostril through which the instrument is to be passed.

The technique of holding the fibrescope depends on the type of instrument available. The *Olympus* type is most widely used in Britain and can be held and operated by either the left or the right hand (Fig. 3.8). The body of this instrument is held by the 2nd, 3rd and 4th fingers and palm and the control knob can then be moved up and down by the thumb. The index finger is placed near the proximal end of the suction channel to seal it for

37

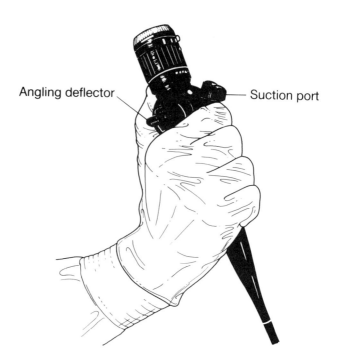

Angling deflector — — Suction port

Fig. 3.8 The fibrescope controls and viewing end as held in the right hand of the operator or The Olympus type of fibrescope.

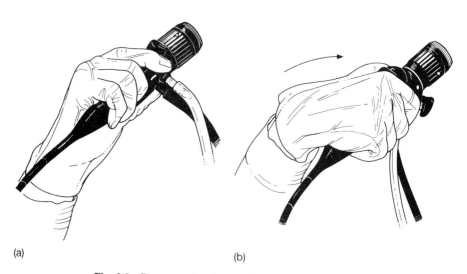

(a)

(b)

Fig. 3.9 Demonstrating the angulation of the bronchoscopists wrist from the normal position in a) to b). This will produce a 180° rotation along the shaft of the fibrescope.

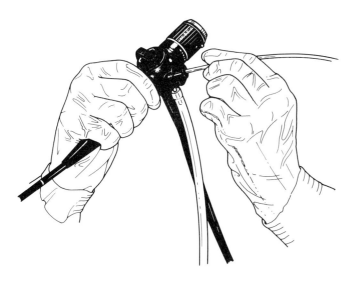

Fig. 3.10 Introducing biopsy forceps or cytology brush into the biopsy channel
of the fibrescope with the (free) left hand.

aspiration as and when necessary. Rotation of the tip is achieved
by rotating the wrist and thus the whole instrument (Fig. 3.9).
The free hand is used to hold steady, advance and withdraw the
shaft as well as to manoeuvre the biopsy forceps and cytology
brushes to their targets (Fig. 3.10). This can greatly reduce nasal
discomfort for the patient.

The *Machida* type of fibrescope is held in the left hand reserv-
ing the right hand to operate the various handles at the proximal
end as well as supporting, advancing and withdrawing the shaft of
the fibrescope. Angulation and rotation of the tip are both
achieved by rotating the proximal eyepiece which twists the distal
end to the right and anti-clockwise twists it to the left. Rotation
can also be achieved by rotating the left wrist.

For all types and makes of instrument the bronchoscope tip is
inserted gently into the nostril under direct vision and passed into
the widest part of the nasal passages. This is usually the inferior
meatus between the inferior turbinate and the floor of the nose.
Lignocaine does not abolish pressure sensitivity and so the bronchoscope should not be forced as this will cause discomfort. The
flexible tip of the bronchoscope is its widest part and once this has
passed through any passage the shaft will follow more easily. If
the bronchoscope will not pass comfortably through either nasal
passage then it should be inserted through the mouth using the
guard as described.

Once the posterior pharyngeal wall is reached the fibrescope is
angulated downwards following the shape of the pharynx and into
the oropharynx behind the uvula. At this stage it should be

possible to see the epiglottis and the glottis in the distance. It may be necessary to aspirate secretions obscuring the view. Care should be taken to ensure that the shaft of the instrument is straight and the patient's chin well forward. Asking the patient to protrude his tongue or to swallow may also help to reveal the epiglottis.

Once the epiglottis has been identified the glottis is usually visible behind and beyond it. If difficulty is encountered in getting behind the epiglottis it may be possible to pass the fibrescope tip laterally and posteriorly alongside the epiglottis and then turn the tip in medially to curl over onto the dorsal surface of the epiglottis. The glottis and the vocal cords are sensitive areas and care should be taken to avoid undue irritation by the bronchoscope tip whilst anaesthetizing this area. Watch for the effects of cardiac dysrhythmias induced by vagal stimulation.

Next, vocal cord mobility should be checked during normal inspiration and expiration by asking the patient to adduct his cords in saying 'see'. Inequality of movement of the cords suggests recurrent laryngeal nerve palsy. The patient should be warned that the next step will cause coughing. This occurs as the vocal cords are anaesthetized by injecting 2 ml of 4% lignocaine (80 mg) onto them in their adducted position via the central channel of the fibrescope.

For purpose of regional anaesthesia via the fibrescope lignocaine should be drawn up as 2 ml aliquots in 5 ml syringes with 3 ml of air in the syringe. The bronchoscope should be positioned with the suction channel uppermost so that the local anaesthetic is injected first and flushed through the central channel by the following air from the syringe.

Two or three minutes are allowed for the lignocaine to have maximum effect and this time should be spent examining the pyriform fossae and the area between the vocal cords and the ary-epiglottic folds. During deep inspiration 2 ml of 2% lignocaine (40 mg) is next injected through the vocal cords into the trachea. The fibrescope tip should be quickly withdrawn a few centimetres during the coughing which will follow. Another 2 ml of the 2% lignocaine is usually required to anaesthetize the trachea adequately.

Before the fibrescope is inserted between the cords into the trachea the patient must be warned that this will make him cough, cause transient breathlessness and that he should not attempt to speak. The patient is advised to resist the impulse to take large breaths but rather to continue with shallow breaths which he should be reassured are sufficient.

During quiet inspiration the bronchoscope is passed gently between the cords through the posterior part of the glottis where the opening is the widest (Fig. 3.11). The patient should be instructed that although the sensation is odd, he can breathe and

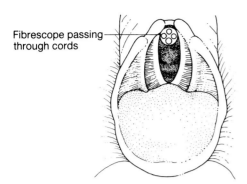

Fibrescope passing through cords

Fig. 3.11 The usual position for the fibrescope between the vocal cords.

swallow normally. A minute or so should be allowed for the patient to become accustomed to the presence of the fibrescope in the trachea. Further boluses of 2% lignocaine may be required if much coughing occurs.

The trachea should be inspected for the appearance of the mucosa and abnormally increased or decreased mobility of the walls should be noted. Similarly the carina should be examined for its sharpness and mobility. Normally the carina becomes shorter and thicker during coughing. Abolition of this variability may indicate infiltration by carcinoma or enlargement of the subcarinal lymph glands.

Further boluses of 2 ml of 2% lignocaine are injected through the suction channel as necessary but the total dose administered should be kept to a minimum by avoiding contact with the bronchial walls thus reducing irritation. If the coughing induced is more than slight it is worth withdrawing the bronchoscope and injecting more lignocaine because once coughing is allowed to become severe it is difficult to control. There is considerable variation in sensitivity of the bronchial mucosa between patients and certainly smokers cough more easily and excessively. Encouragement and keeping the patient informed of what is happening with instructions to keep both eyes open will help to make the examination more comfortable for the patient and easier for the operator.

Both right and left bronchial trees must be systematically examined even if the chest radiograph suggests a unilateral lesion. Opinions vary as to whether the normal or abnormal side should be examined first. It is recommended that the normal side should be inspected first. If examined last it is more likely to be inadequately explored as both patient and bronchoscopist may be tired and secretions and blood may have spilled from the abnormal side following inspection and sampling.

41

Right lung

To examine the *right bronchial tree*, the black notch in the visual field is turned to the right side of the patient. This ensures that the fibrescope tip has maximum manoeuvrability for examination of the bronchi on this side. The *right upper lobe* orifice usually lies just below the carina on the opposite lateral wall; it leads off at an angle of 80–90°. It is helpful to give an extra 2 ml of 2% lignocaine into the upper lobe before it is inspected as the previous doses of lignocaine frequently fail to reach it due to its angulation. The orifice is now entered and the segments and subsegments are examined. The anterior segment which lies ventrally and the posterior segment lying dorsally are relatively easy to inspect without too much manipulation of the fibrescope tip. The apical segmental bronchus is more difficult to enter. To help this manoeuvre, the patient is asked to take a few deep breaths and then to hold the breath at full inspiration when the apical segmental orifice will be more easily seen with the tip of the fibrescope bent maximally upwards towards the head.

The *right middle lobe* bronchus arises ventrally from the intermediate bronchus and extends obliquely downwards. The notch in the visual field of the fibrescope should be placed in the anterior position to aid manoeuvrability in this bronchus which can usually be inspected to subsegmental level.

The fibrescope is then withdrawn back into the intermediate bronchus, the notch rotated dorsally until the orifice of the apical segment of the right lower lobe is seen lying at the same level as the middle lobe. This segmental bronchus branches at 90° from the intermediate bronchus and once again entry into it can be aided by asking the patient to hold the breath in full inspiration.

The remaining segmental orifices of the *right lower lobe* lie several centimetres distal to the apical segment. They all extend downwards and really are an extension of the main bronchus so little difficulty is usually encountered in entering them.

Left lung

After withdrawing the fibrescope back to the carina, the left bronchial tree is next examined by having the notch in the visual field rotated to the left side of the patient. The *left main bronchus* is longer than the right and also deviates more laterally or horizontally in the erect subject. The secondary carina between the upper and lower lobe orifices is a useful landmark.

The lingular bronchus is usually an extension of the upper lobe bronchus and descends downwards dividing into superior and inferior segments.

The upper division of the *upper lobe* bronchus is next examined by withdrawing the fibrescope back into the upper lobe bronchus and turning its tip upwards (headwards) with maximum flexion. This is perhaps the most difficult bronchus to enter. This can be made easier by asking the patient to take a deep breath. The anterior and apico-posterior segments are then examined in turn.

The fibrescope is withdrawn back to the secondary carina and the *left lower lobe* is examined by rotating the notch in the visual field towards it. The apical segmental bronchus arises dorsally almost at the level of the secondary carina. It is located by turning the notch posteriorly and again if difficulty is encountered in entering it, the patient is asked to hold the breath in deep inspiration. The basal segments of the left lower lobe should present no difficulty to examination, noting that the anterior and mediobasal segments are usually combined into a single orifice.

Examination of an average 'normal' tracheobronchial tree has been described. Variations in the branching of the bronchi are frequently encountered and should be borne in mind if apparent abnormalities occur, especially if the mucosa looks normal. At more peripheral levels, individual bronchi or combinations of bronchial orifices cannot be recognized by individual appearances alone because they usually look alike and variations are common. They can only be identified by remembering the route the bronchoscope has taken to get to that point in the bronchial tree. Occasionally it may be necessary to retrace the route to a more central and recognizable bronchus.

A routine of systematic examination of the airways should be adopted to prevent mistakes through omission. In addition to the bronchial tree an orderly inspection of the extrathoracic airways must also be completed. It is valuable to re-inspect bronchi as the fibrescope is being withdrawn to confirm observations made when the instrument was advancing.

Manipulating the fibrescope

The ability to use a fibrescope comes only with practice. Although many useful hints are often given there is no substitute for time spent handling the instrument. The period of time that the novice can spend on a patient is limited and it can be helpful to use the various lung models available. Eventually, operating the instrument should become a subconscious act, like driving a motor car. The experienced bronchoscopist comes to know the position and orientation of the fibrescope tip as a form of extended proprioception, just as a good motorist knows the limits of the front or back of his car. Similarly guiding the instrument with coordinated movements of the wrist, thumb and fingers of the right hand as well as the forward and backward motion of the left hand will begin to occur at a subconscious level.

When this degree of proficiency has been achieved the next problem to overcome is that of manipulating the fibrescope in the patient who will be breathing, moving and coughing. This will obviously require practice and even experienced bronchoscopists continuously improve their technique.

Although the need for practice cannot be overemphasized a few general comments should be useful to the novice. Subject to minor individual variation the best method for holding the fibrescope (Olympus type) is with one hand (the right) with the thumb controlling the 'up–down' lever and the index finger the suction port. The left hand is then free to advance and withdraw the fibrescope at the insertion site or to manipulate the accessory instruments such as the brush or forceps.

Insertion of the fibrescope into the nose or mouth should always be done with the top in the neutral, forward-viewing unlocked position. When advancing the instrument the tip must, as far as possible, always be in the centre of the lumen of the airway. It should be possible to see the whole circumference of the bronchus and avoid scraping the wall. This is achieved by tiny coordinated movements of the right wrist and thumb. Failure to achieve this will cause excess coughing and bleeding. A cycle of coughing once it starts leads to repeated irritation of the mucosa. If this occurs there is no alternative but to withdraw the fibrescope, instill more local analgesic and wait until the coughing stops before advancing again.

Insertion of the fibrescope into segmental or subsegmental bronchi must be done with care. In an average male adult a 5 mm diameter instrument may reach segmental orifices but will be too large to enter them. However, it is often possible to enter subsegmental orifices with a 4 mm diameter fibrescope. Force must never be used to advance or rotate the instrument at any time, paticularly at the segmental and more peripheral levels. Apart from causing trauma to the bronchial wall the angling mechanism of the tip may be damaged. The tactile sensation of increasing resistance to movement of the fibrescope must not be ignored. This readily occurs when the fibrescope is in a peripheral bronchus, the airway distally is magnified as the field of vision of these instruments is up to 100° and their focal range between 3 and 50 mm. It will appear that there is space for the tip to be advanced further, but if this is attempted, the distal bronchus will become 'bunched up' or wrinkled ahead of the fibrescope tip, its orifice will appear to enlarge and it will seem as if the instrument is being withdrawn (Fig. 3.12). If the progress of the fibrescope is felt to be impeded it must be withdrawn even if the airways seems to be large enough. When the bronchial wall is touched the patient will usually begin to cough and this should be heeded.

During fibrescopy, vision is frequently obscured by soiling of the distal objective lens by secretions, pus and blood. Several methods may be used to clean the lens. The end of the fibrescope

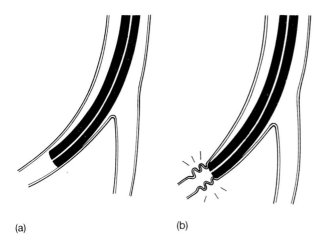

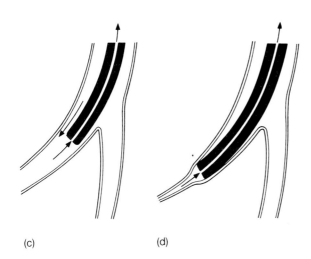

Fig. 3.12 The fibrescope impacted in an airway (a), causing (b) puckering of the lumen. Excessive suction (c) causes the collapse of the distal airway (d).

can be wiped on the bronchial wall or carina while applying suction (Fig. 3.13); the channel can be irrigated with 5–10 ml of saline and then aspirated while the patient coughs. These may clean the lens. If these manoeuvres fail, usually because of adherent blood clot, it is quicker and easier to remove the fibrescope, clean it and reinsert it. Once the vocal cords have been broached it is an easy matter to re-enter them with the fibrescope while the local analgesia is maintained.

Suction is often used indiscriminately because its side-effects are not fully appreciated. If the aspiration pressure is too great the bronchial mucosa is sucked into the fibrescope suction channel

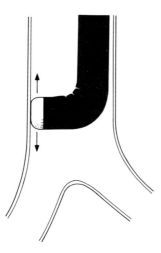

Fig. 3.13   Clearing the tip of mucus or blood by angling it to wipe the distal lens and tip of the fibrescope on the tracheal wall.

and submucosal petechiae may arise even in patients with normal mucosa. In those with mucosa made friable by infection or neoplastic disease, frank bleeding may occur.

Prolonged suction in smaller, peripheral airways into which the fibrescope tip is wedged will cause collapse of the segmental or subsegmental bronchi which have relatively poor supporting cartilage (*see* Fig. 3.12 c & d). With this collapse, spasm of the bronchial wall muscle is liable to follow.

Brisk, intermittent suction is not only more efficient at removing secretions but it also causes fewer side-effects. The pressure of the suction can also be varied by partially covering the hole over the suction channel with a thumb or finger or by turning down the power of the suction apparatus.

SPECIMEN COLLECTION

Much of the value of bronchoscopy depends on the diagnostic yield from accurate specimen collection, preparation and examination. Specimen collection and initial preparation are the responsibility of the bronchoscopist. It is vital that thorough discussion with laboratory staff occurs to establish the optimum methods of specimen collection.

If all possible types of specimens are obtained in every case it should be possible to make the diagnosis in nearly every problem as diagnostic accuracy increases with the number of samples taken. However, time and expense are involved in processing each specimen and only specimens which significantly improve diagnostic accuracy should be undertaken.

The range of specimens needed will vary with the clinical problem and the local range of skilled laboratory services available. Brushings, washings and biopsies are normally required for suspected malignancy and infection whereas transbronchial lung biopsy is needed in diffuse interstitial lung disease. The combination of brush and forceps biopsy produces a high diagnostic yield in bronchogenic carcinoma.

Brush biopsy

Only those types of cytology brushes which have a protective sheath should be used. Brushes with larger bristles give a higher cell yield than those with smaller and more evenly arranged bristles. Old brushes with broken bristles should be discarded and reusable ones should be cleaned carefully between patients to prevent cross-infection and contamination of samples.

If tenacious secretions or blood have been aspirated before brush biopsy, irrigation of the channel with 5–10 ml of saline may first be necessary to avoid extrusion of material in the channel onto the distal objective lens. The brush is held within its polythene sheath which is passed down the suction channel. The sheathed brush is advanced to the required site using repeated short advancing strokes grasping it with thumb and forefinger of the left hand approximately 3 cm from the suction valve. It is positioned above the area for sampling and then an assistant operates the hand control to protrude the brush for sampling. By manoeuvring the tip of the fibrescope the brush is pressed lightly onto the lesion and then advanced and withdrawn several times by pushing the sheath and protruding brush in and out of the suction channel. The assistant then withdraws the brush into its sheath. The sheath and enclosed brush are withdrawn from the suction channel. Sampling of necrotic areas should be avoided as cytology of specimens taken at those sites often proves unhelpful.

Brush biopsy can also be performed on localized peripheral lesions which are not endoscopically visible. Fluoroscopic control of the placement of the brush while not essential, does improve yield. The sheathed brush is inserted into the appropriate segmental bronchus and advanced under fluoroscopic control to the lesion. The position of the brush should be confirmed by turning the patient through 90° or by two-plane fluoroscopy to ensure that the brush does not lie in front or behind the lesion. Brushings are then taken in the usual way. Several bronchi may lead to the area of the lesion and ideally all should be brushed. If the lesion is not visible on fluoroscopy or if fluoroscopy is not available then the brush is advanced to the area which the lesion is seen to occupy on a plain radiograph.

Slides for cytology should be prepared immediately because drying of the specimen in air alters cell morphology making

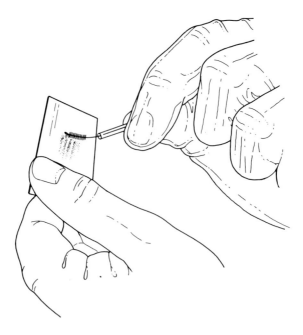

Fig. 3.14 Brush specimen being prepared on a microscope slide.

interpretation difficult or impossible. The bristles of the extended brush are pressed against a clean glass slide and rubbed across its surface (Fig. 3.14). Air-drying is more likely to occur at the edges of the smear and a circular action of the brush on the slide gives better smears than a side-to-side rubbing of the brush against the slide. The diameter of the circular motion should be varied from 0.5–2 cm depending on the amount of cellular material on the brush, i.e. the more material there is, the larger the circle. The critical detail of slide preparation is to ensure that the specimens fixed immediately by alcohol spray or immersion.

An alternative method of handling brush specimens which avoids the problem of air-drying is to agitate the brush in a tube of 0.9% saline solution. This fluid can then be centrifuged in the laboratory and smears are prepared from the sediment obtained. Diagnostic yield by this method is less (70%) than when brushings are transferred directly onto slides.

The ordinary single sheathed brush is inadequate for taking specimens for bacteriological examination because contamination by nasopharyngeal commensal organisms occurs too frequently. Lignocaine should not be injected into the area which is to be sampled as it may inhibit the growth of some bacteria but probably not *Mycobacterium tuberculosis*. Routine brushings should be used in the same way as for peripheral neoplastic lesions. Brushings can then be smeared onto glass slides for appropriate staining and also agitated in saline for culture and subsequent determination of sensitivity to antituberculous drugs.

When infection by agents other than *M. tuberculosis* is suspected a telescoping brush in a double-catheter with a distal plug should be used. This is easier to keep free of contamination by extrathoracic airway commensals (*see* Chapter 4).

Bronchial washings

The simplest and least traumatic method for obtaining specimens for cytology is to instill normal saline through the channel of the fibrescope into the region of the airways under suspicion and then to aspirate into a trap connected in the suction tubing (Fig. 3.15). Such washings are suitable for cytology for malignant disease and for the culture of *M. tuberculosis*.

Usually 5–10 ml of saline is instilled with each wash and about 25–50% of this can be aspirated into the trap. A yield of 5–10 ml of aspirate is usually sufficient for laboratory examination. It is normally convenient to perform brushings before washings, as material which is dislodged by the brush can be aspirated into the trap and at the same time the bronchoscope channel and the bronchus can be cleaned of debris which might obscure vision down the fibrescope. Culturing the trap specimen for bacteria other than mycobacteria is not helpful because contamination with nasopharyngeal secretions occurs in the majority of cases.

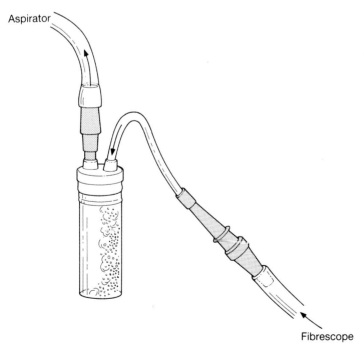

Aspirator

Fibrescope

Fig. 3.15 A suitable suction trap for use with a fibrescope.

Forceps biopsy

Tissue fragments 1–2 mm in diameter can be obtained using fibrescopic biopsy forceps. These small specimens are usually adequate for making a histological diagnosis but sometimes the large biopsies obtained at rigid bronchoscopy may be advantageous. An advantage of the fibrescope is that peripheral and upper lobe lesions are more amenable to biopsy.

Several shapes and sizes of biopsy forceps are available (Fig. 3.16). Smaller forceps, because of their flexibility, are better for

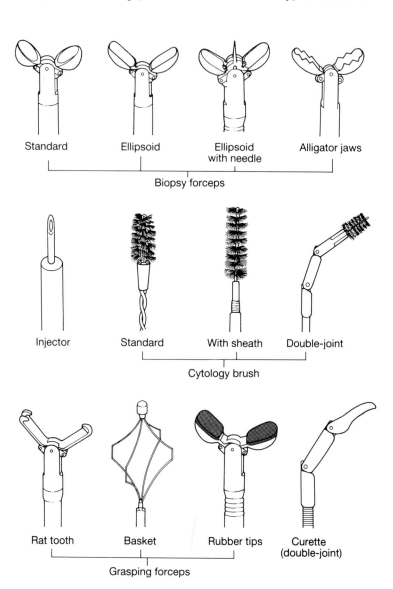

Standard Ellipsoid Ellipsoid with needle Alligator jaws

Biopsy forceps

Injector Standard With sheath Double-joint

Cytology brush

Rat tooth Basket Rubber tips Curette (double-joint)

Grasping forceps

Fig. 3.16 Various biopsy forceps, cytology brushes and equipment for removing foreign bodies and curetting lesions.

taking biopsies from the upper lobes and the apical segments of the lower lobes where the tip of the bronchoscope has to be flexed to an acute angle. Larger forceps can be used for other more easily accessible bronchi.

Before attempting biopsies the channel of the fibrescope should be flushed with normal saline to avoid soiling of the distal lens. While the area of interest is kept in view the forceps are inserted into the biopsy port with the jaws closed. They are then advanced with repeated short strokes by grasping the shaft of the forceps with the finger and thumb of the left hand about 3 cm from the suction valve. Gripping them further away and using larger advancing strokes carry the risk of bending and ruining the delicate forceps control mechanism. When the forceps jaws protrude about 5 mm from the distal end of the fibrescope the assistant is asked to open the jaws and these are advanced onto the lesion and held in place by the bronchoscopist's left hand at the suction valve. The assistant closes the jaws and the biopsy is taken by gently pulling back the forceps until the specimen is removed. Controlled force must be applied in an attempt to cut through the tissue or excessive tissue trauma or damage to the forceps will occur.

The fibrescope tip is returned to the neutral unflexed position and the closed forceps are withdrawn. If the jaws fail to close the forceps cannot be withdrawn. Winding the proximal shaft of the forceps several times round a finger may close the jaws. If this fails the forceps are withdrawn back to the bronchoscope tip under continuous vision and the fibrescope and forceps are carefully withdrawn together.

To prevent damage to the fibrescope the forceps should always be inserted and withdrawn through the channel when the tip is in the neutral or forward viewing position (Fig. 3.17). Attempting to force the forceps through a flexed tip will damage the fibrescope channel and flexing the tip with the forceps jaws in the channel also results in damage to the fibrescope.

After the lesion has been identified and a biopsy has been taken the bronchoscope should be withdrawn to a main or lower lobe bronchus taking note of the path for return to the lesion. The forceps are re-inserted and the bronchoscope is advanced back to the lesion to be biopsied. The presence of the forceps reduces the flexibility of the bronchoscope and it is not always possible to return to the lesion for biopsy. Similarly when the forceps are acutely angled by the fibrescope tip the mechanism of opening and closing the jaws may not work.

Endoscopically visible tumours which are located in line of vision of the fibrescope are not difficult to biopsy but laterally placed lesions on the walls of bronchi are more difficult to sample. For these flexion of the tip of the bronchoscope as far as possible so that the forceps can be jammed against the tumour surface may

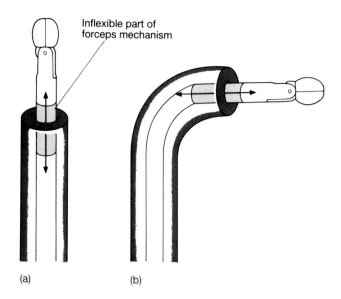

Inflexible part of
forceps mechanism

(a)   (b)

Fig. 3.17 The correct way to insert and withdraw the fibrescope. (a) The inflexible part of the forceps mechanism must be clear of the tip of the fibrescope before angulation and (b) the fibrescope must be restraightened before this portion is withdrawn through the fibrescope.

be necessary. Side-biting forceps (American Cytoscope Makers, Inc.), whose jaws spread to the side when opened are available. Forceps with a central spike with which the lesion can be transfixed before the biopsy is taken may also prove useful (Fig. 3.18).

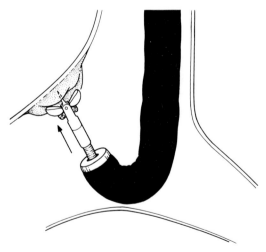

Fig. 3.18 Biopsy forceps with spike for biopsy of lesions on the lateral wall of larger airways.

If previous mild trauma from suction or brushing has produced excessive bleeding, forceps biopsy should not be performed. Vascular tumours, and those with the cherry-red appearance of an adenoma should be biopsied only with caution. Necrotic material often overlies tumours and it may need piecemeal removal with the forceps before a biopsy of histological value can be obtained.

At least three or four good biopsies should be taken and each in turn removed by agitating the open forceps in a small container of 10% formalin. Before reinserting into the bronchoscope the forceps may be washed by agitation in sterile water but this is not essential.

There are several reasons why only small fragments are obtained at biopsy. Firstly the inexperience of the bronchoscopist to whom the biopsies appear large down the fibrescope because of magnification. A common reason is that the assistant applies insufficient pressure to close the forceps fully, however, too much force may break the forceps. Both these problems are remedied by practical experience. Other causes for failure to obtain good biopsies can be that the bronchial mucosa biopsied is normal or the biopsy forceps are blunt.

Occasionally, especially with the large 'alligator' forceps, the bite taken is too big and the biopsy will not come away from the bronchial wall. Excessive force must not be applied, the jaws should be reopened and used to obtain a smaller specimen. Often the plane in which the jaws open is not suitable to take the biopsy. This can be corrected either by rotating the bronchoscope or more easily by rotating the forceps in the channel.

Curette biopsy

When the lesion to be biopsied is in a segmental or subsegmental bronchus it can be biopsied with a curette as in such small bronchi it will not be possible to open the forcep's jaws (Fig. 3.19). The curette is also useful if the lesion lies distal to a bronchial stenosis. The curette head has some mobility as its cutting tip can be flexed to approximately 90° and rotated towards the lesion. The curette is then scraped over the lesion to obtain the specimen. Before withdrawing the tip of the curette it must be straightened to prevent damage to the fibrescope channel lining.

Considerable skill is required to manipulate the curette as it can easily perforate or tear the bronchus. As the curette cuts across a relatively large surface of the mucosa, bleeding occurs more often then with forceps biopsy. These factors limit its usefulness.

Transbronchial lung biopsy

Haemorrhage of 50 ml or more occurs in 49% of patients undergoing transbronchial lung biopsy (TBB). The incidence is higher in

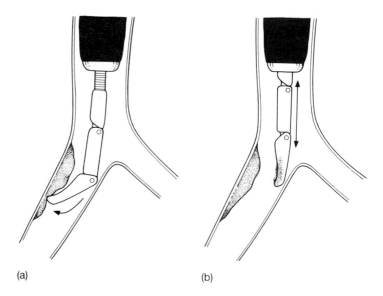

Fig. 3.19 Use of the curette to obtain specimens from lesions on the lateral wall of airways where biopsy forceps cannot be made to impact.

immunocompromised or uraemic patients. For transbronchial biopsy, a clotting screen must be performed and any defects rectified before TBB. The platelet count should be greater than 100 000 and the prothrombin, partial thromboplastin and bleeding times should be normal. The patient's blood group should be known and if the risks seem very high two units of blood should be cross-matched.

At fibrescopy a further safeguard is to take a bronchial biopsy to ensure that abnormal bleeding does not occur. TBB should not be performed in patients with pulmonary hypertension as injury to pulmonary arterioles and capillaries will cause excessive bleeding. Ideally TBB should be performed with fluoroscopic control. In all cases, biopsies should be taken in the region of distal airways as the bronchial and pulmonary vessels also get smaller in size as the airways become smaller towards the periphery of the lung. This reduces the degree of bleeding.

If a peripheral lung lesion to be biopsied is circumscribed, the fibrescope is wedged into the appropriate segmental bronchus as a precaution so that if bleeding does occur it can be confined to that segment. The closed forceps are advanced under fluoroscopy to the lesion and their position is checked by two-plane fluoroscopy or by tilting the patient. The forceps are then withdrawn slightly to allow the jaws to open, readvanced onto the lesion, and the biopsy is taken (Fig. 3.20). The fibrescope is kept in position, wedged in the bronchus, until any bleeding that may have occurred is likely to have stopped. The forceps are withdrawn and the biopsy agitated into a small container of 10% formalin.

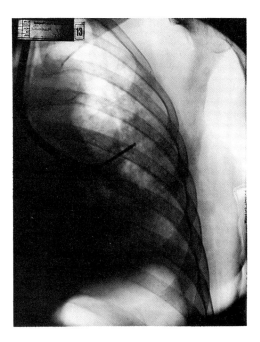

Fig. 3.20 Open biopsy forceps advancing in inspiration to perform transbronchial lung biopsy.

Provided that significant bleeding has not occurred and pleuritic pain has not been caused five or six biopsies should be taken.

The technique for TBB in cases with diffuse lung shadowing on the radiograph is similar. If the disease process appears to be unilateral on radiography the segment with the highest density of shadowing is chosen for the site of biopsy. With bilateral extensive disease the lateral segment of the right lower lobe is selected because the forceps will usually pass to the lung periphery with ease here and little rotation of the patient is necessary to check the forceps position.

The fibrescope is wedged into the selected segment. The closed forceps are passed peripherally under fluoroscopic control into the area of shadowing until they lie about 1 cm from the pleura. They are then withdrawn 1 cm to allow them to be opened more easily in a wider airway. The assistant is asked to open the forceps, and they should be seen to do so on fluoroscopy. The patient takes a deep inspiration as the forceps are then advanced open to within 1 cm of the pleural surface meeting resistance. The patient is asked to breathe out slowly. Towards the end of this expiration the forceps are held gently against resistance from the lung and the jaws are closed. The fibrescope is left wedged in the bronchus and the forceps and the contained specimen are removed. Between four and six specimens are usually taken.

It is generally considered that multiple biopsies are necessary to

55

give a positive diagnosis in diffuse disease as there is thus a greater chance of obtaining an affected, representative piece of tissue. However, Fechner *et al.* (1977) have reported no difference between various pieces of lung obtained with multiple TBB in patients with diffuse lung disease. They found that either all pieces of tissue were diagnostic or none were. If these results are confirmed by other units the practice of multiple TBB should be abandoned.

TBB should always be confined to one lung because of the risk of inducing bilateral pneumothorax.

Specimens of lung obtained by TBB are fixed in 10% formalin. They should be about 2 mm in diameter and float in the fixative indicating that they include alveolar tissue. Occasionally consolidated lung will sink. Inadequate samples are usually due to poor technique or to the forceps being blunt. However, fibrotic lung often yields scanty specimens, presumably because it is less friable than normal lung.

Excessive exposure of the fibrescope to X-ray radiation during fluoroscopy will result in yellow discolouration and darkening of the glass fibre bundles of the fibrescope.

PROCEDURE AFTER FIBRESCOPY

After fibrescopy and specimen collection have been completed, areas of the lungs that have been biopsied are re-examined to ensure bleeding has ceased. The bronchoscope is withdrawn with continuous visualization of the bronchial tree to avoid unnecessary trauma and to confirm earlier observations.

The bronchoscope is cleaned immediately by passing an unsheathed cleaning brush down the channel and then aspirating cleansing fluid through it. The outside of the fibrescope is wiped with gauze soaked in cleaning fluid and is placed in a bath containing a suitable disinfecting solution, some of which is aspirated and held in the biopsy channel by a syringe in the biopsy port.

The patient's recovery will vary with the premedication and sedation used, as well as with any specific investigations that have been performed during the fibrescopy. The effects of local analgesia will remain for up to 2 hours. The patient should be instructed to avoid food or drink during this period and kept under observation by trained nursing staff for 2–3 hours. Vital signs are checked regularly during this period. Supplementary oxygen should be continued in patients with borderline hypoxaemia for up to 12 hours after bronchoscopy.

Some patients, following simple fibrescopy, especially where biopsies have not been taken, are well enough to leave hospital within 1–2 hours of bronchoscopy. They should be discharged after assessment by a physician into the care of a guardian. They are instructed to go directly home and not to take any responsible action, such as driving a motor vehicle, for at least 12 hours. Patients (fit for discharge) who are unaccompanied should be kept under observation longer until they have completely recovered. Patients who are unwell, at special risk, or have undergone TBB should remain in hospital at least over night.

Before the patient leaves hospital some explanations of what was found during the examination and what will happen next must be given. This consultation should be in the presence of an accompanying adult because the amnesic effects of sedation are unpredictable. Instructions and dates of future appointments should be given in writing.

DOCUMENTATION

Correct labelling of specimens, completion of laboratory request forms and the bronchoscopy report are the responsibility of the bronchoscopist. Each specimen must be clearly labelled with the patient's name, date and the site from where the specimen was taken. Relevant clinical details must be provided for the histologist and bacteriologist.

Request forms should be produced in collaboration with laboratory staff and designed to remind the bronchoscopist of the type of information that is required (e.g. diagrams of the tracheobronchial tree on pathology forms). Information about recent chest infections and previous bronchoscopies is vital as these can significantly change the appearance of cells obtained in cytology specimens. Similarly, details of current and recent antibiotic therapy is necessary for appropriate handling of specimens for bacteriological studies.

A bronchoscopy report must immediately provide essential facts on in-patients and urgent cases, with copies to the referring clinicians and for reliable storage and recall. The system used in any unit will depend on the work-load and the facilities available. Simply writing a report in the notes is usually insufficient. At present a system where the bronchoscopist immediately writes the report with a carbon paper copy is simple and convenient. At least three legible copies can be produced by this method. Typing the reports requires a secretary to be present. The advent of microcomputers is likely to change such data storage and handling in the future.

Details of the bronchoscopy report must include the nature and extent of any lesions found with attention to comments on operability of tumours. Diagrams of the bronchial tree are helpful for indicating the siting of lesions and biopsy specimens. Any medication used during or after the procedure must be noted.

57

Brompton Hospital
FIBREOPTIC BRONCHOSCOPY REPORT

Hospital No.

Surname

First Names

D. of B.

M/F

Diagnosis

Ward/dept.

Consultant

Ht.   cm.   Wt.   Kg.   Smoking:

Doctor's Signature   Date

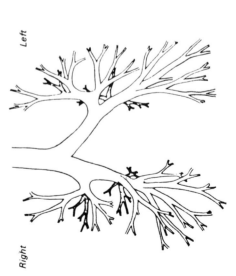

Left

Right

Fig. 3.21 Suitable bronchoscopy report form.

Fibreoptic Bronchoscopy

The extent of the examination and any problems or side-effects are also reported. The report must be signed (Fig. 3.21).

REFERENCES

FECHNER R. E., GREENBURG S. D. & WILSON R. K. (1977) Evaluation of transbronchial biopsy of the lung. *Am. J. Clin. Path.* **68**, 17–20.
GOTHARD J. & BRAITHWAITE M. *Anaesthesia for Thoracic Surgeons*. Blackwell Scientific Publications, Oxford.

4 Diagnostic applications of bronchoscopy

Bronchoscopy became established at the beginning of the 20th Century after the pioneering work of Jackson and Jackson. Initially this important, although limited, procedure was mainly the province of thoracic surgeons who used it primarily to remove inhaled foreign bodies. Chest physicians gradually came to appreciate its usefulness, initially in the management of pulmonary tuberculosis and subsequently in other pulmonary diseases.

With the advent of effective antituberculous chemotherapy, surgical treatment of pulmonary tuberculosis declined and with it the usefulness of bronchoscopy in the management of this disease. Subsequently there has been a marked increase in the incidence of lung cancer and the main role of bronchoscopy today is the diagnosis and assessment of bronchogenic carcinoma.

INDICATIONS FOR BRONCHOSCOPY

The presence of an endobronchial lesion may be suspected on either clinical or radiological grounds. Clinical symptoms and signs may vary from those specific to the respiratory system to those of a more general nature. Thus cough, haemoptysis, wheeze, chest pain or dyspnoea may be present as well as weight loss or clubbing of the digits. Hoarseness, due to recurrent laryngeal nerve paralysis should always be further investigated with bronchoscopy. Abnormal radiological findings such as persistent shadowing of unresolved or slowly resolving pneumonia, hilar or mediastinal abnormalities and diaphragmatic paralysis, may all lead to bronchoscopy. Since the introduction of the fibrescope, with it's low incidence of side-effects and morbidity, it is probably safer to bronchoscope all doubtful cases rather than not.

Cough

Cough is a common symptom and its significance has to be evaluated by considering associated features. It is a normal defence mechanism designed to clear the airways of abnormal material. Tobacco smokers and patients with chronic bronchitis always have a cough and it is these very individuals who are also at most risk of developing bronchogenic carcinoma. An alteration in the character or frequency of cough may indicate new endobronchial pathology, as changes in bowel habit can suggest abdominal neoplasia.

Respiratory tract viral infections are often associated with persistent unproductive cough and the clinician is frequently faced with the decision of whether to perform bronchoscopy with such a history. If the cough persists for 4–6 weeks, then fibrescopy should be performed especially if other risk factors, such as male sex, a smoking history or age 45 years or more are also present.

Haemoptysis

Haemoptysis has been described in association with almost every pulmonary disease as well as in some cardiac disorders and bleeding diatheses. Thus of itself as a symptom it is of little diagnostic value. However, the coughing up of blood is obviously a cause of considerable concern to both the patient and the clinician because it implies serious disease and it may occasionally progress to massive bleeding.

The most common causes of haemoptysis are chronic bronchitis and bronchiectasis, followed by lung cancer and tuberculosis. Haemoptyosis may also occur with pulmonary hypertension, pulmonary infarction, pneumonia, lung abscesses and granulomatous lung diseases such as tuberculosis and rarely sarcoidosis. Brisk bleeding may occur from lung cavities that have become colonized by *Aspergillus fumigatus*.

In general the amount of blood coughed up is rarely of diagnostic value. Lung cancer can present with small or large bleeds although the history is generally of longer than a week. Recurrent small haemoptyses are also a feature of the rare bronchial adenoma.

The mechanism of haemoptysis in patients with chronic bronchitis and bronchiectasis is increased vascularity of the bronchial mucosa. A history of chronic sputum production is usually present. Patients with tuberculosis may present with mild bleeding early in the disease and larger haemoptysis occurs in the later ulcerative phase of tuberculous bronchiectasis, rare now except in Third World countries. It can also result as a recurrent feature of bronchiectatic changes from old but healed disease.

Nasopharyngeal bleeding and haematemesis are not infrequently confused with haemoptysis and, although a carefully taken history can often differentiate between epistaxis, haemoptysis and haematemesis, the upper airway should always be carefully examined at fibrescopy and a subsequent upper gastrointestinal endoscopy will be needed when doubt still exists. Acute pulmonary embolus is an important cause of haemoptysis because

61

it requires prompt diagnosis and treatment which does not usually include bronchoscopy.

Since the advent of fibrescopy, most clinicians would probably agree that all patients with haemoptysis should undergo bronchoscopy except, perhaps, when *M. tuberculosis* is found in the sputum. The purpose of bronchoscopy in these patients is to determine the cause of bleeding, in particular to exclude the presence of cancer, and to identify the site in case of future, unpredictable massive haemorrhage.

The upper airways of patients undergoing bronchoscopy for haemoptysis should be carefully examined. The transnasal route for fibrescopy is ideal as the nasal passages and turbinates can be examined as well as the nasopharynx and oropharynx. All lower airways should be examined systematically to the limits of the visual range of the fibrescope. If no obvious bleeding lesion is found it may be necessary to perform small volume segmental lavages to help identify the source of bleeding. Patients with normal chest radiographs especially require a careful search of all accessible airways.

Bronchoscopy during or within 48 hours of active bleeding is most likely to identify the site of origin of the bleeding. In 120 patients examined during active bleeding with fibrescopy, the site was identified in 93% of cases. Similarly with rigid bronchoscopy the site of bleeding was identified in 86% (18 of 21 cases) in patients who were actively bleeding compared with 52% (41 of 79 cases) examined after the bleeding had stopped (Selecky 1978).

Even when a patient seeks medical advice more than 48 hours after the start of haemoptysis, bronchoscopy should still be performed and if no abnormality is found the patient should be kept under regular review. In a few patients the cause of haemoptysis is never identified but in general most do well. In one study (Selecky 1978) 81 patients with episodes of bleeding which although fully investigated remained undiagnosed were followed up for up to 10 years. In only three patients was the cause later found, and in these it was pulmonary vascular disease. In 10% of patients recurrent episodic haemoptysis continued but without sequelae. In spite of the extremely small possibility of missing cancer or tuberculosis, such patients should be reviewed for at least one year and if haemoptysis recurs they should have a repeat bronchoscopy as soon as possible after the start of new bleeding.

In the presence of massive haemoptysis the immediate danger is acute asphyxiation with aspirated blood. A haemoptysis of more than 600 ml of blood within 24–48 hours has been defined as massive bleeding, but in patients with pre-existing lung disease the respiratory reserve may be so small that even smaller amounts of brisk bleeding may cause respiratory problems. The rate of bleeding is also important. Selecky (1978) reported a mortality of 37% (25 of 67 cases) in patients whose blood loss exceeded 600 ml in 48 hours and 52% (24 of 46 cases) in those who lost similar amounts in 16 hours. For such patients bronchoscopy aims to identify the site of bleeding as quickly as possible. It is vital to maintain an airway and to provide adequate suction so the rigid bronchoscope should be used. Management of massive endobronchial bleeding is described in Chapter 8.

Other symptoms and signs

Partial obstruction of a bronchus may cause a localized wheeze and bronchoscopy may be necessary to differentiate between tumours and other causes of obstruction including endobronchial adenomas or inhaled foreign bodies. All patients with vocal cord paralysis due to recurrent laryngeal nerve palsy or recent diaphragmatic paralysis should be bronchoscoped as well.

Bronchoscopy has been found to be useful in assessing the severity of injury in patients exposed to noxious fumes or smoke. Here bronchoscopic evidence of damage to structures above and below the glottis has proved helpful in management and in predicting the severity of subsequent pulmonary complications.

Bronchoscopy in lung cancer

The clinical presentation of lung cancer is variable. Tumours arising in the lung parenchyma may produce few, if any, signs and symptoms. Small tumours are relatively easily resected and are usually diagnosed by chance on a chest radiograph.

Patients with tumours arising from the main bronchi are likely to present early with cough, haemoptysis, breathlessness and wheeze and in such cases the lesion is usually bronchoscopically visible. The chest radiograph may or may not show abnormalities so that any patient with these symptoms should undergo bronchoscopy or at least sputum cytology.

The bronchoscopic appearance of lung cancer may be directly or indirectly associated with the tumour. The tumour mass itself may be visible or it may be covered by necrotic debris and pus from associated infection as tumour growth outstrips its blood supply. In order to obtain diagnostic histological material, such necrotic material must be cleared before biopsies are taken.

Another direct finding is the appearance of neoplastic infiltration of the surrounding mucosa. This rather vague term encompasses a combination of engorgement of mucosal blood vessels, irregularity of the bronchial mucosa and obscuration of the underlying cartilage suggesting thickening of the submucosa. Similar findings of lesser degree may be present with inflammatory conditions such as bronchitis and tuberculosis. Distinction between the appearance of infiltrating tumour and such already

63

abnormal mucosa may be difficult. Deep biopsies are necessary to give an histological diagnosis in such infiltrating lesions.

The tumour may also indirectly produce endobronchial changes by compressing and distorting the bronchial wall. These changes include stenosis or occlusion of bronchial orifices, narrowing or compression of the bronchial lumen and swelling and erythema of the overlying mucosa. Biopsies taken from such indirect abnormalities are usually not helpful in achieving an histological diagnosis.

If a neoplasm is suspected during bronchoscopic examination cytological and histological material should be obtained to establish the diagnosis. Aspiration of washings, brush and forceps biopsy are the main methods available for obtaining specimens. The diagnostic yield by these various methods depends on the nature of the lesion and the contact made with it. Squamous cell and oat cell bronchogenic carcinomas tend to ulcerate more freely than adenocarcinomas and are more likely to be diagnosed from brushings. If the tumour is small and the bronchus large, brushes and forceps need to be directed with accuracy and this will call for an experienced bronchoscopist.

When the tumour is bronchoscopically visible a histological diagnosis can be made in between 91 and 93% of cases. If the tumour is not visible the positive biopsy rate falls below 45%. Peripheral endobronchial and parenchymal tumours beyond the visual range of the bronchoscope, which can be identified radiologically, can be biopsied using fluoroscopy. Using such fluoroscopic methods a positive biopsy rate of 64% has been claimed but we have been unable to match this. Occasionally, for a variety of reasons, the fibreoptic biopsy may fail to provide tissue diagnosis even when the tumour is visible. Repeat endoscopy is necessary and if the patient is a potential candidate for surgery this might best be left to the surgeon when he makes the final assessment of operability.

Detection of early lung cancer

Early cancer implies limited disease amenable to surgical resection and a good prognosis or even cure. Although it is frequently difficult to determine disease extent before thoracotomy, a useful relationship exists between tumour size and the incidence of lymph node metastases. The incidence of lymph node metastases was shown to be 0.9% in patients with tumours less than 2 cm, and the incidence was 35% for tumours more than 2 cm. The 5-year survival of patients with tumours less than 2 cm was 80% which is significantly greater than for larger tumours (Ikeda 1974).

Ideally all tumours should be detected when they are less than 2 cm in diameter but this is difficult to achieve. Such small tumours on the periphery of the lung can sometimes be identified on chest radiographs. However more central tumours of this size involve large airways where detection is possible by bronchoscopy but at this stage they are usually missed on radiographs. Patients at risk who have symptoms of persistent cough and/or haemoptysis should be bronchoscoped even if the chest radiograph is normal. Because of limited resources at present it is inappropriate to subject at risk patients without symptoms to bronchoscopy as a screening measure. 'At risk' here is defined as over 40 years of age with a smoking history.

Increasingly emphasis has been placed on early diagnosis through sputum cytology and instances have arisen where malignant cells have been found in the sputum but the tumour could not be located on chest radiograph or at bronchoscopy. In such cases a detailed regional study may be performed at bronchoscopy. After a careful fibrescopic search of all segmental bronchi has been made and no evidence of neoplastic disease found, each lobe is brushed in turn with cleansing of the bronchoscope channel and brush between each lobe. Marsh *et al*. (1978) suggested that the lobar bronchus involved can be confirmed in most cases. In one study (King *et al*. 1982) 33 patients whose sputum revealed squamous cell carcinoma with normal chest radiographs were identified. Four other patients had tumour in the upper respiratory tract (one in the nasopharynx and three in the larynx), five more had tumours in the lobar or main bronchus. Of the remaining patients 21 had tumours in a segmental bronchus and in three the site remained unidentified. Several of these patients required two bronchoscopies before the tumour was found.

The importance of careful examination of segmental bronchi must be emphasized when searching for early carcinoma which may appear at bronchoscopy as no more than an area of mucosal reddening or irregularity. Similar appearances can be induced by trauma from the bronchoscope.

At present as an essentially research procedure, fluorescence fibreoptic bronchoscopy has been used to localize small tumours not visible on a chest radiograph. This method is based on the activation of photosensitive material, haematoporphyrin, by ultraviolet light. Haematoporphyrin is taken up preferentially by malignant tissue which then becomes identifiable under ultraviolet illumination. In addition to its diagnostic aspects this substance undergoes a photodynamic reaction on exposure to light which results in cell lysis so that therapeutic applications are being sought (*see* Chapter 5). Disadvantages of this method include the need for expensive laser equipment and photosensitization of the skin which can be a problem, especially in tropical climates, for up to three years after the procedure.

Assessment of operability of endobronchial carcinoma is a vital part of the bronchoscopic procedure.

The extent of the tumour should be defined, in particular with reference to the proximity (in centimetres) of the edge of the lesion to the most proximal carina. Neoplasms involving the main carina or extending onto the trachea are technically inoperable.

Involvement of local lymph nodes and extrabronchial structures can be assessed by observation of the mobility of the bronchial tree during normal breathing, vital capacity breaths and coughing.

If such involvement is suspected or if there are signs of external compression of the trachea, carina or mainstem bronchi it is possible to do a transbronchial needle aspiration biopsy (Fig. 4.1). A long aspiration needle can be inserted via the rigid bronchoscope. The distal 2 cm is of a finer gauge. This can be safely used to penetrate the tracheal wall to aspirate cytology and histology specimens from tumour or involved glands compressing or invading the trachea. Because of the distribution of such glands this method is more often used to sample subcarinal nodes or low, right paratracheal glands. It is not safe to undertake this procedure in the absence of rigidity or compression since normally large blood containing structures, left atrium, pulmonary artery, aorta or azygos vein lie in close proximity to the lower trachea and carina. Recently, considerable success has been reported using this technique with special needle systems developed for fibrescopes.

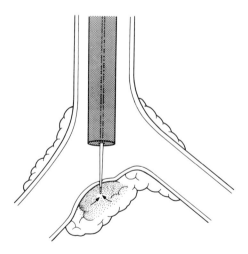

Fig. 4.1 Transbronchial needle aspiration of extrabroncheal lymph glands.

Rigid bronchoscopy assessment

Prior to thoracotomy the surgeon will wish to make his own assessment of a tumour, usually using a rigid bronchoscope. This is especially important if doubt exists as to the resectability of the tumour. Using the rigid instrument under general anaesthesia a precise estimate can be made of the proximal extent of endobronchial tumour, temporarily arresting respiration if necessary. Extrabronchial extension or involved lymph nodes will cause rigidity or compression of the bronchi and subtle degrees of this can be appreciated using the bronchoscope to distort bronchial anatomy. Any doubt remaining as to the extrabronchial spread of tumour will be resolved at mediastinoscopy which should now be routinely used prior to thoracotomy.

Lower respiratory tract infections

In bronchopulmonary infections the contents of expectorated sputum do not necessarily reflect the lower airway flora because of contamination by micro-organisms in the upper airways. Bronchoscopy is a practical and safe method of collecting relatively uncontaminated specimens. This can be of considerable importance particularly in immunocompromised patients in whom the infection may be atypical and severe. Patients commonly presenting with this diagnostic problem include those with leukaemia, lymphoma, autoimmune diseases, following organ transplantation, those on treatment with immunosuppressants and more recently those with acquired immunodeficiency syndrome (AIDS). Fibrescopy can help to identify a variety of organisms including viruses, bacteria and parasites by using the techniques of selective cultures, bronchial washings, bronchoalveolar lavage, brush biopsy and lung biopsy.

Frequently immunocompromised patients are extremely ill and the advisability of subjecting them to invasive investigation may appear questionable. The diagnostic and subsequent therapeutic value of a procedure such as bronchoscopy must be set against the risks of the investigation. The likely outcome of serious and inappropriately treated infection must be carefully evaluated by the clinician. Usually the balance falls in favour of performing the bronchoscopy. Delay in diagnosis may also result in further clinical deterioration of the patient thus making the invasive techniques even more hazardous. It is suggested that in immunocompromised patients with pulmonary infiltrates on chest radiograph, invasive diagnostic techniques should be employed early.

In the critically ill immunocompromised patient certain complications are more likely, and appropriate precautions should be taken. In thrombocytopaenic patients intramuscular injections cause large haematomas and should be avoided. Premedication with intravenous atropine 0.6 mg and pethidine in 25 mg aliquots, sufficient to relieve anxiety, should be used. Lorazepam 1 mg orally 30 minutes before the procedure is better for renal transplant patients as they are often intolerant of narcotics. In patients who are thrombocytopaenic, if the platelet count is less than 1×10^5 a fresh platelet transfusion should be given before bronchoscopy. If adequate arterial oxygenation cannot be maintained, e.g. $(PaO_2 > 80 \, \text{mmHg} \, (10 \, \text{kPa}))$, with supplemental oxygen through an intra-nasal cannula, the patient should have a general anaesthetic and be ventilated with 100% oxygen during the bronchoscopy. Sometimes patients require assisted ventilation before, during and after bronchoscopy.

Specimen collecting procedures

After initial routine insertion of the fibrescope specimen-collecting procedures should be performed in the sequence indicated:
- selective cultures
- brush biopsies
- bronchoalveolar lavage and
- transbronchial lung biopsy

Selective cultures. These are performed by passing a sterile, sheathed brush into the area of infection either, directly when pus is seen, or indirectly into the area of shadowing viewed with fluoroscopic control. Wimberley *et al.* (1979) has suggested that a telescoping double-catheter with a distal plug is not contaminated by upper airway organisms.

For optimum results the following procedure has been recommended by the manufacturers. Topical analgesia should be applied without injecting into the bronchoscope channel, i.e. aerosol or nebulized lignocaine may be used. During the insertion of the fibrescope no topical analgesic should be injected through its channel, nor should any suction be applied, before taking the specimen. This avoids possible inhibition of growth of organisms by lignocaine. If purulent secretions are found the bronchoscope is positioned 4–5 cm proximal to them, if none is found then it is placed in the bronchus of the radiologically abnormal lobe.

The double-catheter unit is inserted into the fibrescope channel and advanced 1–2 cm beyond the bronchoscope tip. The inner telescoping catheter which contains the specimen sampling brush is advanced a further 2–3 cm, which pushes out the protective polyethylene glycol plug (Fig. 4.2). The brush specimen is obtained and the brush is retracted into the inner catheter only; the inner catheter *should not* be pulled back into the outer catheter. The whole brush unit is then removed and the bronchoscopy can proceed normally with topical lignocaine and suction.

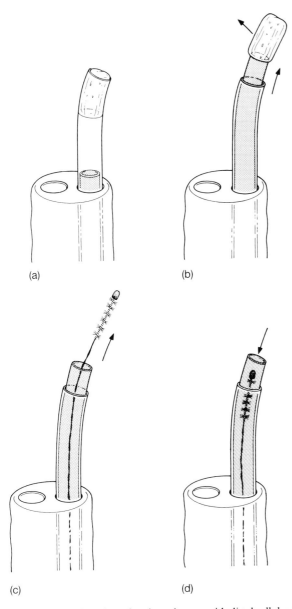

(a) (b)

(c) (d)

Fig. 4.2 Double catheter brush equipment with distal cellulose plug for obtaining uncontaminated specimens for microbiology from the distal airways.

After removal of the double-catheter brush, the most distal part of the inner catheter is cleaned with a sponge soaked in 70% ethanol. The tip of the inner catheter distal to the brush is cut with sterile scissors. The brush is then advanced beyond the new cut end of the inner catheter, taking care to collect secretions pushed out onto sterile glass slides for gram stains. If no secretions are present preparations for microscopy should be made

69

by smearing the brush on to the slides. The brush is then held over a sterile glass pot containing 1 ml of sterile Ringer's lactate solution and cut from the retracting wire with sterile scissors so that it falls into the pot. The pot with the brush is sealed and vigorously shaken. This sample is used for direct plating onto several media, e.g. blood agar, Sabouraud (fungi), MacConkey's (intestinal organisms), Lowenstein–Jensen (*M. tuberculosis*), slopes and tissue cultures (for viruses).

Brush biopsies. Afterwards, routine sheathed brush cytology specimens can be obtained from the affected area using a standard retractable sheathed cytology brush. To obtain the maximum amount of material, the brush should be advanced from its sheath and moved in and out to 'rake' the sample into the sheath which then acts as a collection receptacle. These brush specimens are smeared on to slides and prepared with the following stains: gram (bacteria), Ziehl–Neelsen (*M. tuberculosis*), silver (fungi) and cytological (neoplastic cells and inclusion bodies).

Bronchoalveolar lavage. Bronchoalveolar lavage should be performed in an affected segment preferably other than that from which selective cultures and brush biopsies have been taken. The lavage specimen obtained is divided into two. One part is spun down and slides are prepared from the deposit for examination, as for the brush specimens. The second aliquot is used for preparing the same range of cultures as for the selective brush specimen. The cultures obtained from lavage fluid may be contaminated by nasopharyngeal commensals and the results must be interpreted with care.

Transbronchial biopsy. The diagnostic yield of transbronchial lung biopsy (TBB) in immunocompromised patients with pulmonary infection is high but so is the rate of complications from the procedure and the decision to use it must be considered carefully. If significant bleeding has occurred after brush biopsy TBB is best avoided. Usually three or four biopsies are taken from an area of shadowing in one lung.

Using TBB positive diagnostic yields between 47 and 91% have been reported (Editorial 1983; Willcox *et al.* 1982). *Pneumocystis carinii* pneumonia is particulary amenable to diagnosis by investigation and other opportunistic infections with *Cryptococcus neoformans*, *Aspergillus*, *Phycomycetes*, *Candida albicans*, *Histoplasma capsulatum*, *Coccidioides immitis*, *Blastomyces dermatitidis*, *Torulopsis glabrate*, *Penecillium*, *Nocardia*, viruses, mycobacteria, protozoa and Helminths have all been identified (overall yield 74%) (Ellis 1978).

Various complication rates of transbronchial lung biopsy in immunocompromised patients have been reported. Pneumothorax occurs in between 5.5% and 19% of immunocompromised patients and haemorrhage in 1.3%–26%. The mortality of TBB has been less than 1% (0.2%) but higher than reports for nonimmunocompromised patients. These wide ranges suggest the influence of population differences between reported studies.

In patients with active pulmonary tuberculosis and radiological evidence of disease, diagnosis is sometimes difficult because sputum smears and culture may be negative for *M. tuberculosis*. Several studies have explored the role of fibrescopy in establishing a bacteriological diagnosis. These have shown that in such sputum negative patients an immediate diagnosis (smear positive) can be made in almost 50% of cases and a further 20% give positive cultures. Thus in a prospective 4-year study of 275 patients with suspected pulmonary tuberculosis, 89 (32%) had active disease and in 60 (67%) the diagnosis was made as a result of fibrescopy (Editorial 1983; Willcox *et al.* 1982). Bronchial brushings were positive in 56 patients, 35 on smear and 21 on culture only. Transbronchial biopsies were diagnostic of tuberculosis in nine of 18 patients and this proved the sole confirmation of the bacteriological diagnosis in four cases. Of the remainder another 29 were also considered to have active tuberculosis, the diagnosis being made on the results with post-bronchoscopy sputum, the response to antituberculous chemotherapy or other means. The rest were judged not to have tuberculosis.

Practical problems encountered in bronchoscopy for suspected tuberculosis include the inhibitory effects of local analgesic agents (Conte & Laforet 1962) on *M. tuberculosis* and transfer of infection from one patient to another by the fibrescope (Nelson *et al.* 1983). Lignocaine is the least inhibitory agent but should be used sparingly if specimens for *M. tuberculosis* are being collected. Disinfection of the fibrescope after use with glutaraldehyde for at least 30 minutes or with ethylene oxide is necessary.

Transbronchial lung biopsy in diffuse pulmonary disease

Fibrescopic transbronchial lung biopsy has a place in the investigation of diffuse lung diseases. However, the specimens of lung tissue obtained by this method are small so that accurate diagnosis may not always be attainable. It is possible to obtain larger specimens of lung by transbronchial biopsy with the rigid bronchoscope but again in about 20% of cases there is insufficient tissue, so this method is rarely employed because of its greater morbidity. Tissue specimens adequate for diagnosis have been reported in 80% of patients in one series. The yield of positive histology is less without fluoroscopic control (36–62%) but improves when biopsies are taken from radiologically involved areas of the lung (64–97% positive).

The diagnostic yield also depends on the cause of the diffuse shadowing and is particularly high in sarcoidosis (82%). Yield increases with the stage of the disease from 57% in Stage I, to 77% in Stage II and 91% in Stage III. In conditions where the

71

histological changes vary between different parts of the lung, e.g. fibrosing alveolitis, transbronchial lung biopsy is not so useful and open lung biopsy is preferable to establish the diagnosis and grade the activity of the disease. Conditions where transbronchial lung biopsy gives a high diagnostic rate are lymphangitis carcinomatosa, metastatic lung disease and lymphomatous infiltration of lung. The technique is also of some value in the diagnosis of collagenoses, drug-induced fibrosis and alveolar proteinosis.

REFERENCES AND FURTHER READING

ANDERSON H. A. (1978) Transbronchoscopic lung biopsy for diffuse pulmonary disease: results in 939 patients. *Chest* **73**, 734–6.

CLARK R. A., GRAY P. B., TOWNSHEND R. H. & HOWARD P. (1977) Transbronchial lung biopsy: a review of 85 cases. *Thorax* **32**, 546.

CONTE B. A. & LAFORET E. G. (1962) The role of topical anaesthetic agents in modifying bacteriological data obtained by bronchoscopy. *New Engl. J. Med.* **267**, 957–60.

CUNNINGHAM J. H., ZAVALA D. C., CORRY R. J. & KEIM L. W. (1977) Trephine air drill, bronchial brush and fibreoptic transbronchial lung biopsies in immunosuppressed patients. *Am. Rev. Respir. Dis.* **115**, 213–20.

EDITORIAL. (1983) Fibreoptic bronchoscopy and sputum-negative tuberculosis. *Lancet* **i**, 337–8.

ELLIS J. R. (1978) Diagnosis of opportunistic infections using the flexible fibreoptic bronchoscope. *Chest* **73** (Suppl.), 713–15.

HANSON R. R., ZAVALA D. C., RHODES M. I., KEIM L. W. & SMITH J. D. (1977) Transbronchial biopsy via flexible fibreoptic bronchoscope: results in 164 patients. *Am. Rev. Respir. Dis.* **115**, 780–91.

HERF S. M., SURATT P. M. & ARORA N. S. (1977) Deaths and complications associated with transbronchial lung biopsy. *Am. Rev. Respir. Dis.* **115**, 780–91.

HUNT J. L., AGREE R. N. & PRUITT B. A. (1975) Fibreoptic bronchoscopy in acute inhalation injury. *J. Trauma* **15**, 641–9.

IKEDA S. (1974) *Atlas of Flexible Bronchofibreoscopy*. Igaku Shoin Ltd., Tokyo.

KING E. G., MAN G., LERICHE J., AMY R., PROFIO A. E. & DOIRON D. R. (1982) Fluorescence bronchoscopy in the localisation of bronchogenic carcinoma. *Cancer* **49**, 777.

KNIGHT R. K. (1981) Bronchoscopy and other biopsy techniques. In: Emerson P. (ed.) *Thorac. Med.* Butterworths, London.

KOERNER S. K., SAKOWITZ A. J., APPELMAN R., BECKER N. H. & SCHOENBAUM S. W. (1975) Transbronchial lung biopsy for the diagnosis of sarcoidosis. *New Engl. J. Med.* **293**, 268.

KOONTZ C. H., JOYNER L. R. & NELSON R. A. (1976) Transbronchial lung biopsy via the fibreoptic bronchoscope in sarcoidosis. *Ann. Int. Med.* **85**, 64.

LANDA J. F. (1978) Indications for bronchoscopy. *Chest* **73**, 686–90.

LEFRAK S. S. & TUTEUR F. L. (1977) Transbronchial lung biopsy in diffuse lung disease. *Am. Rev. Respir. Dis.* **115**, 135 (abstract).

LEVIN D. C., WICKS A. B. & ELLIS J. H. (1974) Transbronchial lung biopsy via the fibreoptic bronchoscope. *Am. Rev. Respir. Dis.* **110**, 4–9.

MARSH B. R., FROST J. K., EROSEN Y. S. & CARTER D. (1978) Diagnosis of early bronchogenic carcinoma. *Chest* **73** (Suppl.), 716–17.

MARTINI N. & McCORMICK P. M. (1978) Assessment of endoscopically visible bronchial carcinomas. *Chest* **73** (Suppl.) 718–22.

MITCHELL D. M., EMERSON C. J., COLLYER J. & COLLINS J. V. (1980) Fibreoptic bronchoscopy: ten years on. *Br. Med. J.* **281**, 360–3.

NELSON K. E., LARSON P. A., SCHRAUFNAGEL D. E. & JACKSON J. (1983) Transmission of tuberculosis by flexible fibreoscopes. *Am. Rev. Respir. Dis.* **127**, 97–100.

ROBBINS H. M., MORRISON D. A., SWEET M. E., SOLOMAN D. A. & GOLDMAN A. L. (1979) Biopsy of the main carina: staging lung cancer with the fibreoptic bronchoscope. *Chest* **75**, 484–6.

SELECKY P. A. (1978) Evaluation of haemoptysis through the bronchoscope. *Chest* **73** (Suppl.), 741–5.

SOMNER A. R., HILLIS B. R., DOUGLAS A. C., MARKS B. L. & GRANT I. W. B. (1958) Value of bronchoscopy in clinical practice. *Br. Med. J.* 1079–84.

STABLEFORTH D. E., KNIGHT R. K., COLLINS J. V., HEARD B. E. & CLARKE S. W. (1978) Transbronchial lung biopsy through the fibreoptic bronchoscope. *Br. J. Dis. Chest* **73**, 108–12.

WILLCOX P. A., BENATAR S. R. & POTGIETER P. D. (1982) Use of the flexible fibreoptic bronchoscope in diagnosis of sputum-negative pulmonary tuberculosis. *Thorax* **37**, 598–601.

WIMBERLEY N., FALING L. J. & BARTLETT J. G. (1979) A fibreoptic bronchoscopy technique to obtain uncontaminated lower airway secretions for bacterial culture. *Am. Rev. Respir. Dis.* **119**, 337–42.

5 Therapeutic applications of bronchoscopy

Bronchoscopy allows access to the bronchial tree under direct vision. Thus it may be used to relieve bronchial obstruction and for local application of medications. Foreign bodies are especially amenable to endoscopic removal. Aspiration and removal of thick secretions through the bronchoscope can be helpful in intensive care. Of less value, although it may still have a place, is the bronchoscopic removal of thick or purulent bronchial secretions in acute severe asthma and bronchiectasis. Bouginage of narrowed bronchi may be performed bronchoscopically to relieve localized strictures of the airways.

Therapeutic agents can be applied accurately to bronchial lesions with bronchoscopy. Massive haemoptysis may be controlled by cold saline lavage. Palliative resection of malignant bronchial obstruction may be attempted endoscopically with a cryoprobe, by fulguration or laser therapy. To achieve rather more prolonged effects, radioactive isotopes may be implanted or cytotoxic agents may be injected directly into tumours obstructing major airways.

BRONCHOSCOPIC EXTRACTION OF FOREIGN BODIES

Frequently foreign bodies lodge in major bronchi, especially the right lower lobe and to remove them the rigid bronchoscope is best. Smaller foreign bodies lodged more peripherally in segmental or small bronchi are more easily removed using the fibrescope. Nevertheless, the majority of patients presenting with inhaled foreign bodies are children (94% < 15 years of age) and it is more appropriate to attempt removal with the rigid bronchoscope under general anaesthesia (Cunanan 1978; Holinger *et al.* 1978). It may prove necessary to use the fibrescope as well for the removal of the more peripheral foreign bodies.

The nature of inhaled foreign bodies varies considerably (Fig. 5.1) but the majority are either organic vegetable matter such as peanuts, seeds and pips or sweets. Presenting symptoms and signs usually consist of choking and gagging perhaps followed by a localized wheeze. Organic foreign bodies are often not visible radiologically although the presence of obstructive emphysema on

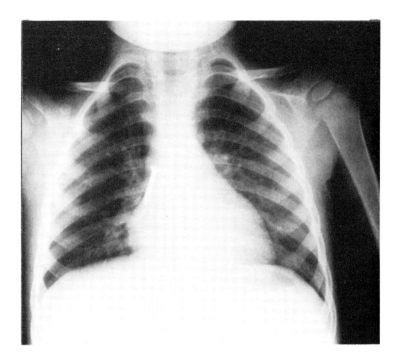

Fig. 5.1 Opaque foreign body on chest radiograph of a child.

an expiration film may help to localize the obstruction. Rarely a non-opaque foreign body may cause more extensive obstructive emphysema and even subcutaneous emphysema by producing a ball-valve obstruction in a main bronchus. Urgent endoscopic removal is indicated to prevent cardiac compression by this 'tension' effect.

Some types of foreign bodies cause particular problems. Inhaled hard 'sweets', such as pear drops or other boiled sweets, produce a thick, sticky material in the bronchus which may require lavage and strong suction to clear. Chewing gum is particularly difficult to remove because it sticks to the mucosa and clogs up the bronchoscope, forceps and suction apparatus. Changes of equipment may become necessary during the same procedure. Dried peas and beans are commonly inhaled by children because they are used in 'pea-shooters'. The initial act in using a pea-shooter is a sharp, deep inhalation with the pea in the mouth. If such a history is obtained, rapid endoscopic removal is advisable as the pea or bean swells on rehydration within the airway and may cause asphyxia within hours.

Foreign bodies removed from older children and adults are more often opaque and may be localized radiologically. These include nails, screws, pins, open and closed safety pins, broken pieces of pens, and teeth. Unfortunately most dental plate fragments are not radiopaque. The main danger of such foreign bodies is that the sharp points and irregular edges may become embedded in the bronchial wall making subsequent extraction hazardous. Biplane fluoroscopy can be useful in such circumstances to help manipulate the foreign body into such a position that the bronchial walls are freed from trauma by the sharp point or edge before attempts are made to extract it.

Practical technique

In the absence of imminent asphyxia, the foreign body should be carefully examined radiologically, in several planes if necessary, to localize it accurately and show it's relation to adjacent structures and the possible position of invisible, non-opaque parts. During bronchoscopy the foreign body should be approached with care in order to prevent pushing it even more distally with the bronchoscope tip. A careful assessment is made of how and where the forceps may be applied to the foreign body.

Various types of special forceps, claws, baskets and balloon catheters are available and it is important to choose the right one and apply it in a good position for successful extraction (Fig. 5.2). The space between the foreign body and the bronchial wall should be examined in order to avoid including the bronchial mucosa with the foreign body when the forceps jaws are closed around it. Occasionally the first application of the forceps may be the best or only opportunity for an accurate, potentially successful grasp at a

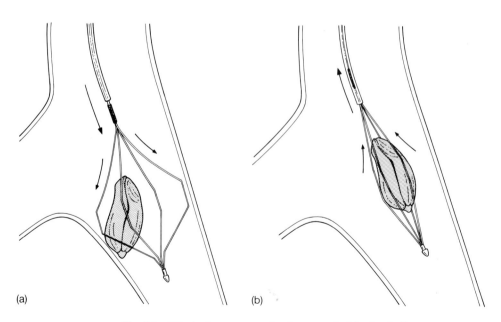

(a)

(b)

Fig. 5.2 Wire basket apparatus for the removal of foreign bodies, e.g. peanut.

peanut or other organic foreign body, for it may fragment and then be irretrievable.

Biplane fluoroscopy has proved useful for the extraction of radiopaque foreign bodies. Objects with sharp points or edges such as open safety pins, can be manipulated under fluoroscopic vision into positions of relative safety before withdrawal. Spherical objects such as ball bearings, or nails and screws with their heads or points proximal may be difficult to grasp unless the forceps blades encompass them beyond their widest diameters. This again is more readily seen with biplane fluoroscopy.

When a firm grasp has been obtained on the foreign body with the forceps or basket the bronchoscope should be advanced towards the foreign body to help release it as the advancing rigid bronchoscope dilates the bronchus. Then the foreign body, forceps and the bronchoscope should be steadily removed together. With the variety of equipment currently available bronchotomy or segmental resection of bronchi are now rarely required to remove aspirated foreign bodies.

BRONCHOSCOPY IN THE CRITICALLY ILL PATIENT

Patients who are critically ill, whether they are being mechanically ventilated or not, frequently have impaired consciousness with depressed cough reflexes and airway clearance. They are particularly prone to retain airway secretions resulting in bronchial obstruction, impaired ventilation and respiratory failure. Physical examination and chest radiography may show areas of collapse-consolidation and routine suction with a catheter may not relieve the obstruction. Here bronchoscopy can often be of considerable use in relieving the airway obstruction and improving ventilation. It should also be considered if aspiration of vomit is suspected.

It has been shown that bronchoscopic clearance of airways is effective in intensive care. In one report of 446 such bronchoscopies 30% of the patients were postoperative and 83% were being mechanically ventilated during the bronchoscopy (Barrett 1978). In 48% of the bronchoscopies retained secretions were found and removed. In almost every case this resulted in improved arterial oxygenation. Radiological atelectasis resolved in 28 of 30 cases and in others retained secretions were found in the absence of radiological abnormalities.

In a study by Stevens *et al.* (1981), 205 therapeutic bronchoscopies were performed in an intensive care unit. Radiological atelectasis was present in 118 cases, most commonly affecting the left lower lobe. Bronchoscopy resulted in radiological and clinical improvement in almost 80% of cases. In 10 patients there was no bronchoscopic abnormality to account for the radiological atelec-tasis but small volume lavage resulted in radiological and clinical improvement in six of the 10.

In these critically ill patients complications of bronchoscopy are impossible to assess, especially when other invasive measures are also used. Hypotension, cardiopulmonary arrest, cardiac dys-rhythmias and mediastinal emphysema have all been reported in association with bronchoscopy.

Fibrescopy can be performed while mechanical ventilation is maintained, but for rigid bronchoscopy it is advisable to change to hand ventilation. A fibrescope with a large suction channel is preferable such as the Olympus BF 1T or Machida 5BS-6TL which have 2.6 mm channels. The Olympus and the Machida 5BS-6TL-W have two channels so that suction and lavage can be performed simultaneously.

The fibrescope is inserted in the standard manner in patients who are not being mechanically ventilated. In patients who have been intubated, the fibrescope is passed down the endotracheal tube provided that this has an internal diameter of 8.5 mm or more. Special adaptors are available to allow the fibrescope to be inserted into the endotracheal tube without producing an air leak but if these are unavailable then a small hole or a slit cut in the rubber sealing section of the endotracheal tube will usually be adequate. Where the endotracheal tube is smaller than 8.5 mm the bronchoscope is passed alongside the endotracheal tube with its cuff deflated. When the fibrescope is in position the cuff is reinflated. To reduce the degree of hypoxaemia 100% oxygen should be administered throughout the procedure.

Aspiration of secretions must always be performed under direct vision. The tip of the fibrescope should just be in contact with the secretions and not with the bronchial mucosa or haemorrhage will occur. If the secretions are beyond the accessible range of the bronchoscope the patient can be asked or made to cough by irritating the mucosa with the bronchoscope tip in order to move the secretions proximally to more central airways. Very thick, tenacious secretions and mucous plugs may be difficult to aspir-ate. Repeated boluses of 3–5 ml of saline injected onto the plugs helps to dislodge them into larger airways where they may be aspirated or coughed up. If no airway obstruction is encountered in the presence of radiological atelectasis, 10–30 ml boluses of saline should be used to 'wash' out the suspect area. Loosened secretions may then become accessible to aspiration. Larger volume lavages probably offer no additional advantage.

Although preferable to the 'blind' use of suction catheters for removing secretions in mechanically ventilated patients, bron-choscopy is obviously not the first step in the management of atelectasis in such circumstances. Routine vigorous chest physiotherapy and 'blind' tracheal suction should be used initially as they are cheaper, less invasive and successful in 60% of cases. If such measures fail then fibrescopy is indicated and, not infrequently, may need to be repeated several times, especially where patients required mechanical ventilation for prolonged periods of time. In centres where fibrescopy is more freely available it has been more readily used. Thus in Japan, 28 of 35 surgical units questioned routinely performed fibreoptic bronchial toilet postoperatively to prevent atelectasis after lung resection (Geddes 1980). The insertion of a flanged tracheal cannula of 4 mm internal diameter through the cricothyroid membrane to produce a minitracheostomy has proved a valuable adjunct to sputum removal following pulmonary resection (Matthews *et al*. 1984). This technique has largely replaced suction bronchoscopy following pulmonary resection, and is now increasingly used in intensive care units to deal with such problems following major surgery or serious illness. This technique has largely removed the need for repeated suction bronchoscopy, but this may still prove necessary as a diagnostic and therapeutic measure if there is persistent lobar or segmental collapse.

Occasionally other uses for fibrescopy in patients requiring endotracheal intubation have been suggested. If intubation is difficult, especially if neck extension is limited, the endotracheal tube can be threaded over the bronchoscope which is then passed into the trachea as an introducer. The endotracheal tube is advanced over it into the appropriate position. If the position of an endotracheal tube is in doubt it can be checked with a fibrescope. Extubation over a fibrescope allows inspection of the trachea, cords and glottis for damage by the tube.

BRONCHOSCOPIC REMOVAL OF ENDOBRONCHIAL MALIGNANCY

Palliative treatment via the bronchoscope can sometimes offer an alternative to radiotherapy for inoperable endobronchial tumour occluding a major airway. Various methods can be used including cryotherapy, fulguration, laser therapy, insertion of radioactive gold grains and local cytotoxic drugs. Of these methods, laser therapy has recently received most attention.

Various forms of palliative therapy can be applied locally to endobronchial tumours via the bronchoscope, avoiding or reducing side-effects which are associated with systemic treatment. Local irradiation can be produced by inserting gold grains into the neoplasm. Cytotoxic chemotherapy can also be injected directly into endobronchial tumours. Direct injections of combinations of cytotoxic agents into all histological types of bronchogenic carcinoma has been shown to lead to bronchoscopic and radiological improvement in all cases and clinical improvement in 18 out of 22 patients (Wagai *et al.* 1982).

Endobronchial gold grain implantation

Radioactive gold grains may be injected directly into endobronchial tumour using an implantation gun attached to a long needle inserted through the rigid bronchoscope. Such radioactive needles may be inserted directly into endobronchial tumour or injected through the bronchial wall into the extrabronchial tumour mass responsible for extrinsic compression. Whilst many techniques are available to deal with the endobronchial component of malignant obstruction it is the extrabronchial component which often proves the most difficult to treat and it is here that endobronchial implantation of gold grains is of greatest value. They may be inserted once other techniques, such as laser endoscopy, have relieved the endobronchial component.

It is ideally suited for patients who have relapsed following external irradiation and where further external irradiation is contraindicated because of the tolerance of normal tissues. Radiation doses in the immediate vicinity of such grains may reach 100 Gray and a total tumour dosage of 60 Gray is frequently achieved. The usual precautions necessary in handling radioactive material must be observed, and such treatment requires the concerted expertise of surgeon, anaesthetist, radiotherapist and physicist. Where there is lobar obstruction, dyspnoea and stridor can be relieved in all patients and 90% will show radiological evidence of reexpansion (Law *et al.* 1985). Improvement is sustained until death in half the patients, but further treatment is feasible in those with recurrent symptoms.

Laser photoresection of endobronchial tumour

Several types of medical lasers have been used including carbon dioxide, argon and the more recent neodymium-YAG. The neodymium-YAG laser is currently the most extensively used and consists of an yttrium-aluminium garnet dotted with neodymium ions.

Several tissue effects can be achieved by laser therapy depending on the power used. At low power (20–40 watts) the light beam is scattered and absorbed in the tissue, and converted into heat. The penetration of the laser beam is about 5 mm, the heat produced evaporates the water in the tissue and coagulates the blood in the vessels. The tissues shrink and can be removed with biopsy forceps. At higher power levels (60–80 watts) the superficial tissue is vaporized and so much energy is used up in this process that little penetrates to surrounding tissue. The depth of tissue thus affected by higher power is usually less.

The success achieved by Dumon *et al.* (1984) is due partly to their technical expertise based on a current experience of more than 1504 laser treatments on 839 patients and partly to careful selection of patients for such therapy. On this impressive series the mortality rate was only 0.3%. All six deaths occurred during the postoperative period, five being due to cardiovascular arrest, infarction or anoxia (not defined) and one to haemorrhage. Immediate reversible complications included bradycardia (three cases), cardiac arrest or collapse (four cases), haemorrhage greater than 250 ml (14 cases), pneumothorax (three cases) and emphysema (one case). Endobronchial fire and penetration of the bronchial wall were not encountered.

Dumon *et al.* (1984) recommended the use of a rigid broncho-scope for all but low-grade obstruction or peripheral lesions, as better control of the airway and haemorrhage can be achieved with the rigid instrument. A rigid bronchoscope specially designed for laser therapy is now used (custom-made Wolf bron-choscope). This has two ports, one for the laser fibre and one for the suction catheter with an adaptor for treatment under closed circuit anaesthetic methods. If necessary another catheter can be passed down the main bronchoscope channel. A disadvantage of this technique is that general anaesthesia is usually required for rigid bronchoscopy and this may not be possible in patients with extremely poor respiratory reserve. But fewer treatment sessions, usually only one or two, are required with the rigid system because it is undoubtedly more effective as more tumour tissue can be removed at one session.

The majority of serious complications appear to occur in the postoperative period. Careful observation of the patient close to the endoscopy unit is advisable. Problems including retained secretions, haemorrhage from loosened necrotic tissue and bron-chial perforation from delayed tissue necrosis can all cause hypox-aemia, and repeat bronchoscopy may be necessary. Bronchial perforation may result in damage to a large artery and further laser therapy in such cases may be ineffective in stemming the bleeding.

The laser beam can destroy submucosal tissue without affecting the surface and the effectiveness of the treatment may not be apparent for several days until this tissue has sloughed off. More often, endobronchial manipulation can cause mucosal swelling so that the tumour boundary cannot be identified and the procedure has to be abandoned. Although rare, fire has been reported during laser resection, produced by the presence of heat and combustible materials. This is preventable by using low power settings below 45 watts to allow adequate cooling of the laser tip and by not administering an inspired oxygen concentration greater than 50%.

A small but recognized risk to the endoscopist and other personnel in proximity to the laser is that of the laser beam, even after many reflections, hitting the eye, causing punctiform retinal destruction. Care must be exercised when handling the equipment and protective goggles must be worn throughout. It must be appreciated that the wave-length of the neodymium-YAG laser is in the infra-red spectrum and therefore invisible to the human eye.

Although the immediate results of laser therapy may be impressive, it is palliative treatment only. Most endobronchial tumours spread extensively into the lung parenchyma and their true extent cannot be assessed endoscopically. Central inoperable tumours causing respiratory difficulty due to airway obstruction are amenable to this therapy producing temporary relief of obstruction.

It is extremely rare that a central inoperable tumour can be identified early enough for complete resection by laser therapy. A new method of localizing and treating early carcinoma has been introduced and although still experimental, it has interesting possibilities. This method is based on the activation of photosensitive material by light. The photosensitizing agent has an affinity for malignant tissue and on exposure to light undergoes a chemical reaction which causes cell death. The photosensitizer currently used is a haematoporphyrin derivative (HpD) and a red light source is administered with an argon laser at least 48 hours after an intravenous injection of the sensitizer. Although showing some promise the results of this expensive form of treatment are, as yet, limited. A recognized side-effect of this therapy is photosensitization of the skin which may cause burns on exposure to sunlight for some 2–3 years after the treatment.

REFERENCES AND FURTHER READING

BARRETT C. R. (1978) Flexible fiberoptic bronchoscopy in the critically ill patient. *Chest* 5, (Suppl.), 746–9.

BRUTINEL W. M., CORTESE D. A., & McDOUGALL, J. C. (1984) Bronchoscopic phototherapy with the Neodymium-YAG laser. *Chest* 86, 158–9.

CASEY K., FAIRFAX W., SMITH S. & DIXON J. (1983) Intratracheal fire ignited by the Nd-YAG laser during treatment of tracheal stenosis. *Chest* 84, 295–6.

CORTESE D. A. & KINSEY J. H. (1984) Hematoporphyrin derivative phototherapy in the treatment of bronchogenic carcinoma. *Chest* 86, 8–13.

CUNANAN D. S. (1978) The flexible fiberoptic bronchoscope in foreign body removal: experience in 300 cases. *Chest* 73, (Suppl.), 725–6.

DUMON J. F., SHAPSHAY S., BOURCEREAU J., CAVALIERE S., MERIC B., GARBI N. & BEAMIS J. (1984) Principles for safety in application of Neodymium-YAG laser in bronchology. *Chest* 86, 163–8.

FEISELMAN J. F., ZAVALA D. C. & KEIM L. W. (1977) Removal of foreign bodies (two teeth) by fibreoptic bronchoscopy. *Chest* 72, 241.

FISHER J. (1983) The power density of the surgical laser beam: its meaning and measurement. *Lasers Surg. Med.* 2, 301–15.

FOREHAM D. R. (1977) Palliative endobronchial implantation of radioactive gold seeds. *Am. Rev. Respir. Dis.* 115, 107.

GEDDES D. M. (1980) Fibreoptic bronchoscopy in the intensive care unit. *Intensive Care Med.* **6**, 145–6.

HAYATA Y., KATO H., KONAKA C., AMEMIYA R., ONO J., OGAWA I., KINOSHITA K., SAKAI, H. & TAKAHASHI, H. (1984) Photoradiation therapy with hematoporphyrin derivative in early and Stage I cancer. *Chest* **86**, 169–77.

HETZEL M. R., MILLARD F. J. C., AYESH R., BRIDGER C. E., NANSON E. M., SWAIN C. P. & WILLIAMS I. P. (1983) Laser treatment for carcinoma of the bronchus. *Br. Med. J.* **286**, 12–16.

HODGKIN J. E., ROSENOW E. V. & STUBBS S. E. (1975) Oral introduction of the flexible bronchoscope. *Chest* **68**, 88.

HOLINGER P. H. & HOLINGER L. D. (1978) Use of the open tube bronchoscope in the extraction of foreign bodies. *Chest* **73** (Suppl.), 721–4.

LAW M. R., HENK J. M., GOLDSTRAW P. & HODSON M. E. (1985) Bronchoscopic implantation of radioactive gold grains into endobronchial carcinomas. *B. J. Dis. Chest* **79**, 147–51.

MATTHEWS H. R. & HOPKINSON R. B. (1984) Treatment of sputum retention by minitracheotomy. *B.J.S.* **71**, 147–50.

MILLEDGE J. S. (1976) Therapeutic fibreoptic bronchoscopy in intensive care. *Br. Med. J.* **4**, 1427.

OHO K., HARUBUMI K., OGAWA I. & AMEMIYA R. (1981) Present status of bronchoscopy in Japan. *Br. J. Dis. Chest* **75**, 409.

STEVENS R. P., LILLINGTON G. A. & PARSONS, G. H. (1981) Fibreoptic bronchoscopy in the intensive care unit. *Heart lung* **10**, 1037–45.

WAGAI F., KINOSHITA M., SHIRAKI R. & WATANABE, H. (1982) The direct injection of several anti-cancer drugs into the primary lung cancer lesion through a fibreoptic bronchoscope. *Nippon Kyobu Shikkiu Gakkai Zasshi* **20**, 170–5.

WAYAND W. (1979) Controlled clinical trial 'blind' versus aimed fibrebronchoscopic suction in mechanically ventilated patients. *Anaesthetist* **28**, 92–6.

Therapeutic applications

6 Paediatric bronchoscopy

Bronchoscopy is less frequently undertaken in the child since the major indication in the adult is related to long standing acquired disease associated with cigarette smoking. The expertise is best concentrated in the hands of a few individuals and varying from area to area this service may be provided by a chest physician, an ENT surgeon, a general paediatric surgeon, or a thoracic surgeon. The indications for bronchoscopy in the neonatal, infant and paediatric age groups are:

1   stridor
2   persistent wheeze or cough
3   haemoptysis
4   persistent or recurrent atelectasis/consolidation
5   obstructive emphysema
6   prior to bronchography to clear the secretions and to check the bronchial anatomy
7   where there is the remotest possibility of foreign body.

It is concern as to this last possibility which partly underlies many of the other indications for bronchoscopy.

In most respects bronchoscopy in children is similar to that in adults. There are however important differences dictated by the smaller calibre of the airways in children. The sections which emphasise these differences are:

• equipment
• anaesthesia
• technique
• postoperative care

EQUIPMENT

The small calibre of the child's airway restricts the endoscopist to the use of narrow bronchoscopes with little facility for additional instrumentation. Present fibreoptic equipment is relatively bulky, and if made small enough for the child permits no channel for biopsy or suction. Fibreoptic equipment is ideal for laryngoscopy, but for more extensive examinations of the tracheobronchial tree the rigid instrument is still routinely used by the majority of endoscopists. A range of instruments is manufactured by Stortz. These instruments have proximal lighting using a prism so that light rods do not further reduce the field of vision. The child's head is relatively large and therefore the upper airways are long in comparison with that of adults. To negotiate these airways the bronchoscope must be proportionally longer than the adult instrument. Most manufacturers produce instruments only 20 cm in length, but longer instruments can be obtained and are recommended. As the diameter of the instrument increases so there is an increase in the range of instruments which may be passed, increasing the therapeutic and diagnostic value of the examination.

The Stortz 2.5 instrument has an outside diameter of 4.5 mm with an internal diameter of approximately 3 mm. This instrument is ideal for premature infants and neonates. It is wide enough to allow the passage of a fine 2.8 mm forward viewing telescope to allow examination of the distal airways. The instrument can also accommodate a suction catheter, but biopsies must be taken without the aid of the telescope using tiny biopsy forceps.

The size 3 instrument is available in 20 cm or 26 cm lengths, and the latter is preferred. The external diameter of this instrument is 5 mm with an internal diameter of 4 mm. This instrument may be used on children age one month to a year. This instrument allows the passage of an optical biopsy forcep attached to the telescope so that small biopsies may be taken under direct vision. With the 3.0 and 2.5 size instruments foreign body removal must be undertaken using a foreign body basket, and although this ingenious instrument aids removal it remains a difficult procedure as the guide wire considerably reduces the field of vision. Fortunately foreign bodies are unusual in children below the age of one year.

For a child older than one year the size 3.5 bronchoscope can be used and it is available in 26 cm length. The instrument has an external diameter of 5.5 mm and an internal diameter of almost 5 mm. In addition to the instruments available with the smaller bronchoscopes, this instrument will also accommodate an optical foreign body forcep attached to the telescope. This greatly facilitates foreign body removal.

The larger instruments, size 4 and 5, may be used in larger children, but the increase in size is no longer so critical as a full range of instruments may be used through either bronchoscope. The size 5 bronchoscope is available in 30 cm length and has an external diameter of 8 mm and an internal diameter of 6.5 mm. It is satisfactory for children of 5–6 years or older. It is clearly best to use the largest instrument which may be passed through the larynx without trauma and a range of instruments should be available at each examination.

General anaesthesia is used routinely for paediatric and infant bronchoscopy since these patients are unable to co-operate sufficiently under local anaesthetic. Preoperative medication is optional; in addition to providing sedation it may be desirable to prescribe an antisialogogue (e.g. atropine 0.01 mg/kg) to reduce oropharyngeal secretions. If suxamethonium is to be the neuromuscular blocker chosen then the administration of atropine preoperatively or at induction is mandatory to counter-act its vagal effects.

Traditional anaesthetic techniques for paediatric bronchoscopy use deep inhalational anaesthesia with oxygen and ether or oxygen and halothane. This technique allows the anaesthetist to defer inserting a venous line until the child is asleep. However, its disadvantages are inevitable periods of hypoventilation and hypoxia, cardiovascular depression and the slow emergence from anaesthesia. An alternative and now more common technique uses intravenous induction, for instance with thiopentone (3–5 mg/kg). Neuromuscular blockade is then established with sux-amethonium (1 mg/kg initially and increments of 0.5 mg/kg to a total of 3 mg/kg) for short procedures, or a non-depolarizing neuromuscular blocker such as atracurium (0.4 mg/kg) for pro-cedures in excess of 15 minutes or in patients in whom post-operative ventilation is considered inappropriate.

Ventilation may be maintained either using a Venturi technique or by the use of a ventilating sidearm on the bronchoscope. The snug fit of the bronchoscope within the child's airway at once makes ventilation with the venturi more hazardous and facilitates ventilation by the sidearm. If the latter technique is to be used an eyepiece must be fitted to the proximal end of the bronchoscope. A simple slide is available which allows the proximal opening to be occluded by the eyepiece or by a perforated cap which main-tains positive pressure ventilation during the passage of the telescope (Fig. 6.1). This slide also has a large open port for the passage of biopsy forceps and other larger instruments, but these may temporarily impair ventilation. An advantage of this tech-nique is that the system allows inhalational anaesthesia to be maintained with ease. Should a Venturi technique be selected there is a theoretical argument that positive pressure ventilation using the Venturi system is more likely to dislodge a foreign body into the distal airways. However, since foreign bodies are rela-tively firmly placed this argument is probably overestimated. Care must be taken to select an appropriate calibre of injector needle in the range of 18–20 standard wire gauge to prevent barotrauma which may produce surgical emphysema or air embolism in thin walled airways.

At the termination of the examination the instrument is

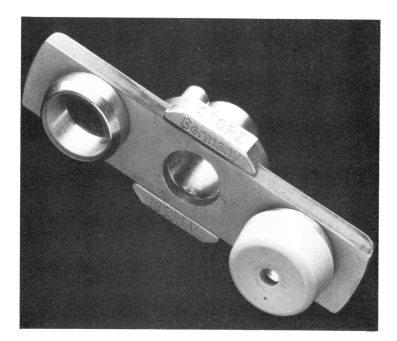

Fig. 6.1 Details of sliding eyepiece.

replaced by an endotracheal tube which allows more accurate
assessment of the return of spontaneous ventilation. The endotracheal tube may be required to be left in place until upper airway
oedema, due to mechanical causes, has settled.

TECHNIQUE

Because of the child's relatively large head it is necessary to
extend the neck and head by inserting a sandbag beneath the
shoulders so that the larynx is visualized. An assessment of
laryngeal size is made using an intubating laryngoscope and the
appropriate bronchoscope is introduced between the vocal cords.
Because of the small calibre of the airways any oedema, particularly of the vocal cords, will cause a disproportionate amount of
airway obstruction. The endoscopist must ensure that too large an
instrument is not passed and the consequent limitations on endoscopic manoeuvres must be accepted. Intubation past the larynx
must be with extreme care and any unnecessary movement of the
instrument from side to side or up and down the trachea avoided.
Using the small instruments, examination beyond the trachea
should be undertaken with the telescope. In larger children the
bronchoscope may be passed into the main bronchi but again a
greater proportion of the examination is completed using the
telescope than is usual in adults. The flexibility of a child's airway
permits a good view of the upper lobe bronchi using a straight

87

viewing telescope. As with adults a careful systematic examination should be made, identifying all segmental branches. The biopsies obtained are similar in size to those produced with the fibreoptic instrument. Any bleeding produced must be cleared completely as this, like oedema, will have a disproportionate effect on airway patency.

POSTOPERATIVE CARE

Following bronchoscopy children require careful monitoring to detect stridor which may occur several hours after the examination. During this time the child must remain in a well staffed high dependency area with trained paediatric nurses, medical staff and an anaesthetist always available. Should there be any hint of stridor developing, humidification should be given via an oxygen mask or head box. The child should stay in this safe area until all stridor is resolved.

7 Research application of bronchoscopy

Fibreoptic bronchoscopy affords a direct means of access to the bronchial tree, and is safe and well tolerated by most patients. In consequence it is possible to study regional or local anatomy and physiology in health and disease. Regional lung function can be investigated by selectively intubating segments or even subsegments of the lung. Local gross anatomy can be directly visualized. By taking mucosal or transbronchial lung biopsies histology can also be examined. By lavaging lung segments, viable cells can be obtained so that cellular mechanisms can be studied *in vitro*.

REGIONAL LUNG FUNCTION

Patients with lung disease confined to a segment, or even a lung are often considered for surgical resection of the diseased area. Indeed, for patients with bronchial neoplasm, surgery provides the only possibility for cure. When other tests have shown no evidence of metastatic disease, surgery is performed if the respiratory function of the lung tissue that is not to be resected is adequate for survival. Routine, non-invasive physiological lung function studies are invaluable for preoperative assessment but they provide information of the total lung function. In some instances it is of considerable importance to distinguish between the relative contribution of diseased and normal parts of the overall lung function. This can in part be assessed on the chest radiograph and ventilation/perfusion lung scans. Assessment of regional lung function can identify inoperable patients more accurately and the diseased part may be shown to be a significant contribution to overall lung function. Conversely, if it can be demonstrated that the affected lung is serving no useful function, then patients with relatively poor lung may not be denied surgery.

By intubating the bronchial tree, information about regional lung function can be obtained at the segmental, lobar or individual lung level. The concept is not new, and bronchospirometric techniques have been used in man since the introduction of the double-lumen rigid bronchoscope in 1932. The function of the right and left lung was separately assessed using this technique. However, the instrument was awkward to use and unpleasant for the patient and so was soon abandoned.

Interest in regional lung function was transiently rekindled in the late 1940s by the introduction of flexible twin-lumen catheters for bronchospirometry, which could distinguish between right and left lung function. Subsequently a triple-lumen catheter was developed which allowed the right upper lobe to be studied separately from the remainder of the lung. Although these methods were used as research tools, the associated morbidity and mortality precluded their widespread clinical application.

Following the introduction of the respiratory mass spectrometer in the late 1950s, the possibilities for measuring regional lung function were once again considered. Elegant methods involving the catherization of lobar bronchi with fine stainless steel mass spectrometer sampling tubes were developed for use at rigid bronchoscopy. Various indices of regional lung function were measured using these techniques in dogs. Clinical applications were again not explored because of the poor acceptability by patients of rigid bronchoscopy under local analgesia, and the limited availability of mass spectrometers.

Fibreoptic bronchoscopy has provided an acceptable method for intubation of the bronchial tree to the segmental level under local analgesia. Currently, various techniques are being developed to assess different aspects of regional lung function using fibrescopy.

Static lung volumes of parts of the lung can be estimated with a radioactive tracer gas and subsequent planimetry of the gamma camera record. The inspiratory gas is labelled with [81]krypton directed down the channel of the fibrescope during a slow inspi-

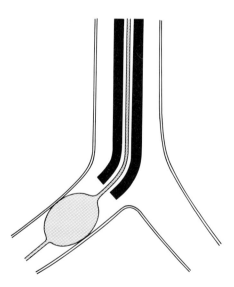

Fig. 7.1 A balloon catheter procluding the right main bronchus.

ration. With the fibrescope positioned in the orifice of the lobe or segment this technique can be used to determine the size, shape and position of each segment or lobe of the lung. Anterior and lateral views of the segments are obtained and volumes for each can then be estimated. Observations on the redistribution by cardiac beat mixing of a marker gas during a breath-hold, the effects of convection and slow inspiration can also be made by this technique.

Before the advent of the fibrescope regional dynamic lung volumes could only be assessed in patients sedated sufficiently to allow the introduction of large endobronchial tubes. Patients undergoing flexible bronchoscopy are only lightly sedated so that they are able to co-operate with the breathing procedure involved in spirometry. The fibrescope is placed in the appropriate lung, lobe or segment and a balloon catheter is passed down the suction channel (Fig. 7.1). The balloon is inflated to occlude the part of the lung under examination and spirometry of the remainder and the trapped part can be studied separately at the mouth. Thus values for PEFR, FEV_1 and FVC can be obtained for both diseased and unaffected regions of the lung.

Clinical applications

Measurement of regional lung function in the preoperative assessment of bronchogenic carcinoma has not yet been extensively studied by these bronchoscopic techniques. Bagg and Cox (1984) have recently described a method for determining regional lung function by balloon occlusion of the bronchus to the lobe or lung to be resected using a Fogarty balloon catheter introduced at fibrescopy. They demonstrated a significant correlation between preoperative prediction of postoperative vital capacity and FEV_1 and the actual values measured at follow-up after surgery.

Single-breath Argon-Freon tests have been used to estimate regional ventilation and perfusion in patients with bullous lung disease and poor overall lung function being considered for surgery. Of 22 patients tested, 10 were recommended as suitable for surgery on the basis of these regional results (Waller 1982). Routine lung function tests such as static and dynamic lung volumes and carbon monoxide transfer characteristics were similar in those considered suitable for surgery and those not suitable. Of the 10 patients, six underwent surgery: four lobectomy and two a modified Monaldi procedure. Five of these surgical patients reported subjective improvement in dyspnoea postoperatively. Routine postoperative lung function in all six showed significant reductions in hyperinflation with no change in carbon monoxide transfer capacity, suggesting that poorly venti-lated and poorly perfused lung had been removed.

These initial clinical studies indicate that such regional studies may have a part to play in the assessment of localized lung disease. These bronchoscopic techniques need to be compared for clinical usefulness, side-effects and patient tolerance with less invasive methods for the assessment of regional function such as radio-isotope imaging, computed tomography and nuclear magnetic resonance.

BRONCHOALVEOLAR LAVAGE (BAL)

The use of bronchoalveolar lavage in the study of immune mechanisms at the airway and alveolar level stems from the idea that the cellular and noncellular material washed out by this procedure will be a representative sample of the contents of the lower respiratory tract. Whether this is valid is debatable, but at least in theory the bronchial tree offers a means by which samples of inflammatory and immune material can be obtained from healthy and diseased lungs.

An experimental lavage procedure was used successfully by Myrvik *et al.* (1961) to obtain pulmonary macrophages from lungs of rabbits. Subsequently Harris *et al.* (1970) used a Metras bronchographic catheter to isolate and lavage the lower lobes of volunteers who reportedly tolerated the procedure well and good samples of macrophages were obtained. Not until the introduction of the bronchofibrescope was this pioneering work further developed and the research and clinical applications of BAL are still being defined. With the fibrescope, this procedure can be performed with little risk and minimal discomfort to the subject.

Methods

Minor modifications of the basic technique for instillation and aspiration of saline in the lung exist, and different institutions tend to adopt their own regimens. These minor variations may affect the results and the incidence of side-effects. It is therefore important to standardize the procedure so that results between centres can be compared. Patients with suspected interstitial lung disease (usually cryptogenic fibrosing alveolitis or sarcoidosis) frequently undergo BAL as a part of their assessment. Contra-indications to BAL include:

1 current heart disease
2 $FEV_1 < 1$ litre
3 resting arterial oxygen tension $70 < $ mmHg (9 kPa)
4 age > 65 years

Pre-lavage investigations should include a chest radiograph and lung function tests including arterial blood gas estimations. Written, informed consent should be obtained from all patients.

Routine fibreoptic bronchoscopy under local anaesthesia is

performed. Supplementary oxygen is administered with a single nasal catheter to the unoccupied nostril in an attempt to counter-act the transient hypoxaemia which invariably occurs following lavage.

The bronchoscope is wedged into a segmental bronchus, the standard site being the lateral segment of the right lower lobe, and 180 ml of saline, corrected to pH 7.4 by the addition of a calculated volume of sodium bicarbonate (BP 8.4%, 275 μl/500 ml of standard 0.9% physiological saline) and prewarmed to 37°C, is introduced. The bronchoscope is disimpacted and the fluid is aspirated into a silicon lined glass bottle using a suction pressure of between 200–400 mmHg to avoid mucosal trauma. If the recovery volume is >100 ml, the procedure is terminated; if not, lavage is continued in sequential 60 ml aliquots to reach a total of 100 ml of recovered fluid, stopping at a maximum of 360 ml fluid introduced whatever the volume recovered.

The recovered lavage sample is transported immediately on ice to the laboratory for examination. Oxygen administration is con-tinued for 2 hours following the lavage through a Ventimask (35%).

The procedure adopted by Hunninghake *et al.* (1979) at the National Institute of Health Bethseda, differs in minor details. Here the bronchoscope is wedged into the subsegmental bronchus of the lingula or right middle lobe rather than the lower lobe. Aliquots of 20 ml of 0.9% sterile saline are inserted and immedi-ately aspirated with a suction pressure of 50–100 mmHg. This process is repeated five times so that total introduction volume is usually 100 ml. Occasionally up to 300 ml of fluid may be inserted if recovery of fluid is poor or if a larger sample is required. During the aspiration procedure the bronchoscope is kept firmly wedged in the segmental bronchus.

Side-effects

Hypoxaemia due to fibreoptic bronchoscopy is well recognized (*see* Chapter 8). Lavage in addition to bronchoscopy causes an increase in the degree of hypoxaemia induced (Fig. 7.2). This can be reduced with supplementary oxygen therapy during the proce-dure. The wedging of the fibrescope and the instillation of the lavage fluid cause ventilation/perfusion inequality resulting in hypoxaemia.

The physiological effects of lobar lavage with saline have been investigated in healthy, non-smoking human volunteers. Unfor-tunately, the results obtained in normals are not directly compar-able with those from patients undergoing this procedure, because method used in that study differed from ones normally used in patients. In the healthy volunteers 10 × 100 ml aliquots of saline (total 1 litre) were instilled whereas most patients normally

93

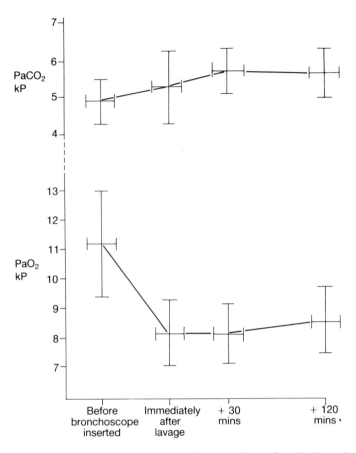

Fig. 7.2 Arterial oxygen and carbon dioxide tensions before, during and after bronchoalveolal lavage.

receive less than 300 ml (Burns *et al.* 1983). However, the results may be comparable in that the patients have lung disease and thus greater prior susceptibility to hypoxia.

Of the 19 volunteers, 13 had lavages and six were 'sham' controls. All 19 developed hypoxaemia (PaO_2 80 mmHg, 11 kPa) because ventilation to the lobe to be lavaged was prevented by a cuff on the bronchoscope. Supplemental oxygen (15 l/min by mask) reduced but did not eliminate this hypoxaemia. The degree of hypoxaemia was significantly greater in the group undergoing lavage compared with controls.

[133]Xenon ventilation and perfusion scans demonstrated both ventilation and perfusion abnormalities in all 19 subjects. These abnormalities had resolved within 2–4 hours in the control group but persisted up to 24 hours in the lavaged subjects, two of whom developed infiltrates on chest radiograph in lobes other than those lavaged. The perfusion defects were less and cleared more rapidly in those on supplemental oxygen.

Respiratory function tests were performed before and 2–4 hours after lavage. A 20% fall in total lung capacity occurred after lavage with saline at room temperature, but this was not apparent if saline at body temperature was used. Residual volume was increased and small airways resistance (as measured by the FEF 25–75) was increased by lavage. FEV_1, VC (vital capacity), and FRC were not altered.

Four lavaged subjects, but none of the controls, developed a pyrexia >38°C which resolved within 24 hours. All the subjects tolerated the procedure well and no significant or irreversible problems were encountered. A mean of almost 80% of the instilled fluid was recovered.

The nature and frequency of side-effects of BAL encountered in patients have been reported in a few studies. Cole *et al.* (1980) reported the complications of BAL on 120 patients with recurrent acute respiratory infections, fibrosing alveolitis or carcinoma of the bronchus. Six consecutive patients had serial arterial blood gas estimations during and after lavage. A mean fall in arterial oxygen (PaO_2) of 3.0 kPa (22.7 mmHg) was found but no significant change occurred in $PaCO_2$. The PaO_2 remained low for 2 hours after lavage. Eight of 42 patients studied prospectively with a four-hourly record of temperature and a chest radiograph at 24 hours, developed fever and six of these also had abnormal radiographic shadowing. These complications resolved quickly with antibiotics and physiotherapy. Three of the 120 patients had unspecified respiratory distress which resulted in termination of the procedure, and a similar number developed pallor, loss of consciousness, bradycardia and hypotension during or immediately following BAL. All patients recovered without sequelae.

Strumpf *et al.* (1981) reported a lower incidence of side-effects. They performed 281 BAL procedures over a 3-year period on 119 individuals with interstitial lung disease and 22 normal volunteers. No mortality or major complications were encountered but 5% of the procedures were associated with minor problems. The most frequent complication was postlavage fever which occurred in seven patients (2.5%). This resolved without therapy in six and one patient received penicillin. Bleeding due to traumatic insertion of the bronchoscope occurred in two patients but this resolved spontaneously. Bronchospasm developed in one patient and resolved after bronchodilator therapy. The low incidence of side-effects reported in this study may be due to the relatively small lavage volumes used (100–150 ml), but unfortunately neither the incidence nor the magnitude of these side-effects can be compared with other reports because definitions of fever and bronchospasm were not given.

A more recent retrospective study by Dhillon *et al.* (1986) reports a higher incidence of minor side-effects in 170 BAL procedures on 104 patients with interstitial pulmonary diseases.

Again no major complications were encountered. Postlavage pyrexia as defined by a rise in oral temperature $>1°C$ occurred after 26% of procedures. Lavage volumes of 180–360 ml were used and a positive correlation between an increasing incidence of pyrexia and increasing lavage volume was demonstrated. Treatment with prednisolone and immunosuppressive drugs was associated with a higher incidence of pyrexia. The postlavage pyrexia resolved spontaneously within 24–48 hours in the majority of patients, only seven (4%) required antibiotic therapy. Other side-effects included bradycardia in two patients (1%) and haemoptysis in one (0.6%). A fall in PEFR of >20% was noted after 24% of procedures and three patients (2%) required bronchodilator therapy. However, a similar incidence (23%) of fall in PEFR was found to occur after bronchoscopy without BAL and it was concluded that this was not an effect of the lavage.

These reports conclude that BAL in patients with interstitial lung diseases is a safe procedure and is associated with only minor, transient side-effects which are acceptable to both the patient and the clinician, especially in relation to the value of the information made available by this technique.

Application

At present the use of BAL as an aid to diagnosis and management in various lung diseases is still being evaluated, and clear guidelines for the use of the technique have not as yet been formulated, although useful information has been made available in interstitial fibrosis by this means. The range of materials obtained from the fluid and cells from normal lungs has been extensive but standardization of methods is essential before valid comparisons with disease states can be made.

Samples obtained by performing BAL on segments or subsegments are at present considered to be representative of the lung as a whole. It has been proposed that the cells and proteins recovered with BAL accurately reflect those present in lung parenchyma.

REFERENCES AND FURTHER READING

BAGG L. R. & COX I. D. (1984) Balloon occlusion of the bronchi at fibreoptic bronchoscopy: application to physiological assessment before lung resection for bronchogenic carcinoma. *Thorax* **39**, 236.

BJORKAMN S. (1934) Bronchospirometric, eine Klirnsche methode, die function der menschlichen lungen getrenut und gleichzeitig zu untersuchen. *Acta. Med. Scand.* **56** (Suppl. 82), 1–199.

BURNS D. M., SHURE D., FRANCOZ R., KALAFER M., HARRELL J., WITZTUM K. & MOSER K. M. (1983) The physiologic consequence of saline lobar lavage in healthy human adults. *Am. Rev. Respir. Dis.* **127**, 695–701.

CANDER L. & FOSTER R. E. (1959) Determination of pulmonary parenchymal tissue volume and pulmonary capillary blood flow in man. *J. App. Physiol.* **14**, 541–5.

CARLANS E. (1949) A new flexible double-lumen catheter for bronchospirometry. *J. Thorac. Surg.* **18**, 742–6.

COLE P., TURTON C., LANYON H. & COLLINS J. (1980) Bronchoalveolar lavage for the preparation of free lung cells: technique and complications. *Br. J. Dis. Chest.* **74**, 273–8.

DENISON D. M. & WALLER J. F. (1982) Interpreting the results of regional single-breath studies from the patients' point of view. *Bull. Europ. Physiopath. Resp.*, **18**, 339–51.

DHILLON D. P., HASLAM P. L., TOWNSEND P. J., PRIMETT Z., COLLINS J. V. & TURNER-WARWICK M. (1986) Bronchoalveolar lavage: side-effects and factors affecting fluid recovery. *Europ. J. Respir. Dis.* **68**, 342.

FOWLER K. T. & HUGH-JONES P. (1957) Mass spectrometry applied to clinical practice and research. *Br. Med. J.* **1**, 1205–7.

GEE J. B. L. (1980) Editorial: Bronchoalveolar Lavage. *Thorax* **35**, 1–8.

HARRIS J. O., SWENSON E. W. & JOHNSON J. E. (1970) Human alveolar macrophages: comparison of phagocytic ability, glucose utilization and ultra-structure in smokers and nonsmokers. *J. Clin. Invest.* **49**, 2086–96.

HASLAM P. L., TURTON C. W. G., HEARD B. *et al.* (1980) Bronchoalveolar lavage in pulmonary fibrosis: comparison of cells obtained with lung biopsy and clinical features. *Thorax* **35**, 9–18.

HUNNINGHAKE G. W., GADEK J. E., KAWANAMI O., FERRANE V. J. & CRYSTAL R. G. (1979) Inflammatory and immune processes in the human lung in health and disease: evaluation by bronchoalveolar lavage. *Am. J. Pathol.* **97**, 149–206.

JACOBAENS H. C., FRENCKNER P. & BJORKMAN S. (1932) Some attempts at determining the volume and function of each lung separately (bronchospirometry). *Acta. Med. Scand.* **79**, 174–215.

MYRVIK Q. N., LEAKE E. S. & FARISS B. (1961) Studies on pulmonary alveolar macrophages from the normal rabbit: a technique to procure them in a high state of purity. *J. Immunol.* **86**, 128–32.

PIERCE R. J., BORWN D. J. & DENISON D. M. (1980) Radiographic, scintigraphic and gas-dilution estimates of individual lung and lobar volumes in man. *Thorax* **37**, 773–80.

STRUMPF I. J., FELD M. K., CORNELIUS M. J., KEOGH B. A. & CRYSTAL R. G. (1981) Safety of fibreoptic bronchoalveolar lavage in evaluation of interstitial lung disease. *Chest* **80**, 268–71.

WALLER J. F. (1982) *Assessment of a Single Breath Test of Whole and Regional Lung Function in Man.* MD thesis, University of London.

WEINBERGER S. E., KELMAN J. A., ELSON N. A., YOUNG R. C. Jr. REYNOLDS H. Y., FULMER J. D. & CRYSTAL G. (1978) Bronchoalveolar lavage in interstitial lung disease. *Ann. Intern. Med.* **89**, 459–66.

WEST J. B. & HUGH-JONES P. (1959) Effect of bronchial and arterial constriction on alveolar concentrations in a lobe of the dog's lung. *J. Appl. Physiol.* **14**, 743–52.

WILLIAMS S. J., PIERCE R. J., DAVIES N. J. H. & DENISON D. M. (1979) Methods of studying lobar and segmental function of the lung. *Br. J. Dis. Chest.* **73**, 97–112.

WILLIAMS S. J., PIERCE R. J., DAVIES N. J. H. & DENISON D. M. (1979) Methods of studying lobar and segmental function of the lung in man. *Br. J. Dis. Chest.* **73**, 97.

ZAVALA D. C. & HUNNINGHAKE G. W. (1983) Lung Lavage. In: Flenley D. C. & Petty T. L. (eds) *Recent Advances in Respiratory Medicine*, pp. 21–33. Churchill Livingstone, London.

8 Complications of bronchoscopy

Bronchoscopy is a safe procedure if a thorough assessment of the patient is first made and appropriate precautions are taken. It is mostly well-tolerated if performed by an experienced, sympathetic bronchoscopist. It must be recognized that infrequent serious complications can occur even under the most favourable circumstances.

Patient assessment should include a careful history and physical examination. Specific enquiries for detection of special risks are advisable e.g.:

1 with a history of asthma, bronchoscopy may result in bronchospasm

2 bleeding diatheses may give excessive bleeding when biopsy specimens are taken

3 patients with renal failure are especially prone to profuse haemorrhage

4 postbronchoscopy infection may occur in patients who are immunocompromised

5 superior vena caval obstruction predisposes to laryngeal oedema and persistent bleeding after bronchoscopy

6 cardiac dysrhythmias and ischaemic heart disease are relative contraindications to bronchoscopy and it should be delayed at least six weeks after a myocardial infarction.

Some degree of airways obstruction and hypoxaemia occur during bronchoscopy and this persists immediately afterwards.

Routine investigations that have been recommended prior to bronchoscopy have included:

1 spirometry: FEV_1 and FVC

2 chest radiograph

3 haemoglobin estimation and full blood count

4 urea and electrolytes

5 electrocardiogram

6 arterial blood gases

7 hepatitis type B antigen

8 clotting screen: prothrombin time
                 partial thromboplastin time
                 platelet count
                 (bleeding time)

Previous drug allergies should be noted, especially to drugs that are likely to be used in the premedication and anaesthesia, so that they can be avoided. Current medication with anticoagulants and cardiorespiratory depressants may need to be temporarily stopped.

INCIDENCE AND NATURE OF COMPLICATIONS

The morbidity and mortality associated with bronchoscopy are generally considered to be low and few reports have been published for almost 10 years. Credle, Smiddy & Elliott (1974) published a review of a questionnaire answered by 192 physician fibrescopists. They reported a total of 24 521 bronchoscopies of which 8378 were performed either through an endotracheal tube or a rigid bronchoscope and 3850 had general analgesia. Complications were considered minor if not life-threatening, required no resuscitative therapy and caused no lasting morbidity, the rest were deemed to be major.

A total of 110 complications were encountered (0.45%); 30 were attributed to the premedication or anaesthetic and 80 to the bronchoscopy. Three patients died (0.01% mortality): one death was ascribed to local anaesthesia and two to the bronchoscopic procedure itself.

Premedication accounted for 13 complications, nine minor and four major. These were respiratory depression, transient hypotension, syncope and 'hyperexcitability'. Premedication should be kept to a minimum and if possible not used at all in patients who have low respiratory drive, e.g. with chronic respiratory failure.

A total of 17 complications of local anaesthesia were noted, six minor, 10 major with one death. These included respiratory arrest, convulsions, cardiovascular collapse, laryngospasm and methaemoglobinaemia. The agent tetracaine was the cause in seven cases, including the one death. This is currently not used, having been replaced by the safer lignocaine. Even with lignocaine the margin of safety is small and the total dose must be kept to a minimum, wherever possible the total dose should not exceed 400 mg.

Of the 80 complications of the bronchoscopy itself, 67 were minor, 11 major and two patients died. Laryngospasm was the commonest problem (31 cases) and was usually induced by attempts to pass the fibrescope between inadequately anaesthetized vocal cords. Bronchospasm occurred in six cases and two of these required resuscitative bronchodilator therapy. Other complications of bronchoscopy were respiratory compromise (nine), syncope (one), cardiac arrest (one), other cardiac dysrhythmias (10), postbronchoscopy fever (eight), pneumonia (two) and epistaxis (12).

The results of this study should be interpreted with some caution because of its retrospective multicentred nature. That the incidence of complications was underestimated is suggested by Pereira *et al.* (1975), who prospectively investigated 100 patients undergoing fibrescopy for fever, and pneumonia. A 16% incidence of postbronchoscopy fever and a 6% incidence of pneumonia was noted. Increased age and abnormal endoscopy findings were considered to be significant predisposing factors.

Hypoxaemia during fibrescopy

Any instrument introduced into the respiratory tract will cause obstruction to airflow, increase airway resistance and so affect respiratory gas exchange. The fibrescope invariably causes airflow obstruction because it is a solid instrument with a narrow suction/biopsy channel through which little air can pass. Thus resistance to airflow at a flow rate of 0.5 l/s with an endobronchial tube of 8.5 mm internal diameter in place is approximately 2 cm $H_2O/l/s$. With a 4 mm fibrescope inside the endotracheal tube the resistance increases to about 7 cm $H_2O/l/s$, and with a 6 mm fibrescope to 20 cm $H_2O/l/s$. This obstruction to airflow results in some degree of hypoxaemia in most patients. The resting PaO_2 has been shown to drop by an average of 2.5 kPa (20 mmHg) during fibrescopy and the fall in PaO_2 increases with the duration of the procedure, and lasts up to four hours after bronchoscopy (Albertini 1975).

The rigid bronchoscope causes little obstruction because it is an open tube and as the procedure is usually performed under general anaesthesia, ventilation with a Venturi system can be matched to requirements.

Abnormalities of cardiac rhythm during fibreoptic bronchoscopy have been demonstrated by continuous ECG monitoring. In 50 patients studied prospectively, major cardiac dysrhythmias occurred in 40% of patients (Katz 1981). Ventricular dysrhythmias occurred in 20% of patients and were found to be most frequent during the insertion of the bronchoscope through the vocal cords. Continuous monitoring of arterial oxygen saturation showed that hypoxaemia appeared to be the main factor contributing to these cardiac dysrhythmias. No correlation was found between the frequency of dysrhythmias and the patients' age, sex, premedication or pre-existing cardiac or pulmonary disease. No adverse clinical sequelae resulted from these ECG abnormalities so that, apart from the occasional patient with severe cardiac disease, it appears that routine ECG monitoring of patients during fibreoptic bronchoscopy is not necessary.

Supplementary oxygen should probably be administered to all patients undergoing fibrescopy and is mandatory for all patients in whom the resting arterial oxygen tension is 9 kPa (>70 mmHg) or less. A single nasal catheter into the nostril not used for the fibrescope is convenient and practical. A 40% Venturi mask modified by cutting a 2 cm diameter hole in its side and fitting the hole with a thin rubber diaphragm containing a slit through which the fibrescope is passed, is effective in maintaining oxygenation but is more cumbersome. Supplementary oxygen should be continued for at least two hours after the procedure in those patients previously known to be hypoxic.

Complications of transbronchial lung biopsy (TBB)

Problems associated with the biopsy procedures of fibrescopy are often discussed but except in specific circumstances, such as the biopsy of an adenoma, their incidence and severity has rarely been calculated.

Complications associated with TBB have been reported but the experience of each bronchoscopist has been small so that an accurate incidence of problems is not available. The incidence of disabling pneumothorax after TBB is generally considered to be about 2% and major haemorrhage 0.3% provided that appropriate screening and precautionary measures have been taken.

In a report of 5450 TBB's (Herf & Suratt 1978) pneumothorax occurred in 5.5% and was the most frequent complication; one patient died from a tension pneumothorax. Usually the pneumothorax develops directly after the biopsy procedure but can occur many hours later especially if the patient is being mechanically ventilated. A routine expiration chest radiograph is advisable after all TBB procedures and patients should be observed carefully for at least 12 hours.

Significant haemorrhage (greater than 50 ml) occurred in 1.3% and accounted for nine deaths. Eight of the deaths occurred in patients who were known to have disorders of coagulation because of their disease or therapy.

There are several methods which may be employed to control haemorrhage. Vision will be obscured even by small amounts of bleeding onto the objective lens of the fibrescope and locating the source of bleeding will be almost impossible. Immediate treatment consists of localizing the bleeding to a lobe or lung and increasing inspired oxygen concentration to the blood-free lung while trying to stop the haemorrhage.

Before a TBB is taken the fibrescope should be wedged into the segmental or lobar bronchus and the instrument is kept wedged for 2–3 minutes after the biopsy. Thus if bleeding does occur, it will be confined to the segment or lobe. Prior instillation of a 5 ml bolus of 1:20 000 adrenaline into the segment selected for lung biopsy may help to reduce the amount of subsequent bleeding.

Moderate amounts of blood can be aspirated via the fibrescope channel and if bleeding continues the supplementary oxygen should be increased and an intravenous infusion started to maintain the blood pressure.

If these initial measures fail to control the bleeding a Fogarty catheter (No. 4) can be passed down the fibrescope channel into the bronchus and inflated with 0.5–1.75 ml of radiocontrast (Hypaque) if available, or saline. The proximal end of the Fogarty catheter is then clamped and the plastic hub cut off. A straight plug is inserted into the catheter to maintain the pressure in the inflated balloon and the clamp is then removed. The fibrescope is carefully removed over the catheter, cleaned and can be reinserted beside the Fogarty catheter to aspirate blood and secretions proximal to the inflated balloon. The inflated catheter can be left in position until the bleeding has stopped (Gotlieb & Hillberg 1975).

If massive haemorrhage remains uncontrolled the fibrescope should be left in the bleeding bronchus on continuous suction and the patient turned so that the bleeding side is dependent. Help should be summoned from an anaesthetist and a thoracic surgeon as soon as possible. The next step is to insert a rigid bronchoscope to aspirate the blood and tamponade the bleeding bronchus. Another method is to isolate the non-bleeding lung with an endobronchial tube or a Fogarty occlusion catheter (8–14°F, 80 cm long with 10 ml balloon) (Gourin & Garzon 1975).

Similar methods are used to control bleeding from peripheral tumours but it is not possible to isolate centrally located lesions. In these cases, if brisk haemorrhage occurs which cannot be aspirated sufficiently quickly through the fibrescope, the instrument should be removed, the patient turned with the bleeding side dependent and a rigid bronchoscope inserted to aspirate the blood more quickly.

In these circumstances the patient will become agitated further increasing blood loss. Sedation with opiates or diazepam will be valuable and general anaesthesia is often required.

PATIENT ACCEPTABILITY OF FIBRESCOPY

Patients' tolerance for fibrescopy under local anaesthesia appears to be good. Studies of patients' subjective experience of fibrescopy, have shown that in the usual uncomplicated procedure most of the patients' discomfort arises from fears and anxieties, the effects of premedication and injudicious comments by the bronchoscopist and helpers (Bernard 1983).

In another study of fibrescopy under local anaesthesia 60 patients completed a questionnaire about discomfort during the procedure. Only 18% found the experience very unpleasant whilst the majority found it mildly unpleasant (55%) or not unpleasant

(27%) (Johnson *et al.* 1978). Approximately 45% of patients noted Complications
pain mostly in the nose (37%) or pharynx (20%) and infrequently
in the larynx (8%) or trachea (3%) (Johnson *et al.* 1978).

REFERENCES AND FURTHER READING

ALBERTINI R. E., HARRELL J. H. & MOSER K. M. (1975) Management of arterial
hypoxaemia induced by fibreoptic bronchoscopy. *Chest* **67**, 134–6.

BERNARD J. (1983) Bucking Broncho. *Spectator* 9 July 1983: **31**.

CREDLE W. F., SMIDDY J. F. & ELLIOTT R. C. (1974) Complications of fibreoptic
bronchoscopy. *Am. Rev. Resp. Dis.* **109**, 67–72.

EDITORIAL. (1974) Safety and fibreoptic bronchoscopy. *Br. Med. J.* **4**, 542–3.

GOTLIEB L. S. & HILLBERG R. (1975) Endobronchial tamponade therapy for
intractable haemoptysis. *Chest* **67**, 482.

GOURIN A. & FARZON A. A. (1975) Control of haemorrhage. *Chest* **68**, 120–1.

HERF S. M. & SURRATT P. M. (1978) Complications of transbronchial lung
biopsies. *Chest* **73** (Suppl.), 759–60.

JOHNSON N. McI., HODSON M. E. & CLARKE S. W. (1978) Acceptability of
fibreoptic bronchoscopy under local anaesthesia. *Practitioner* **221**, 113–14.

KARETZKY M. S., GARVEY J. W. & BRANDSTETTER R. D. (1974) Effect of
fibreoptic bronchoscopy on arterial oxygen tension. *NY State J. Med.* **1**,
62–3.

KATZ A. S., MICHELSON E. L., STAWICKI J. & HOLFORD F. D. (1981) Cardiac
arrhythmias: frequency during fibreoptic bronchoscopy and correlation with
hypoxaemia. *Arch. Intern. Med.* **141**, 603–6.

KNIGHT R. K. (1981) Bronchoscopy and other biopsy techniques. In: Emerson
P. (ed.) *Thoracic Medicine*. Butterworths, London.

PEREIRA W., KOVNET D. M., KHAN M. A., IACOVINO J. R., SPIVACK M. L. &
SNIDER G. L. (1975) Fever and pneumonia after flexible fibreoptic bronchoscopy. *Am. Rev. Resp. Dis.* **112**, 59–64.

PERRY L. B. (1978) Topical anaesthesia for bronchoscopy. *Chest* **73** (Suppl.),
691–3.

ZAVALA D. C. (1978) *Flexible Fibreoptic Bronchoscopy*. University of Iowa, Iowa.

9 New hazards of bronchoscopy

The standards of cleanliness used for fibreoptic bronchoscopy have changed progressively with time. When the technique was first introduced most bronchoscopies were carried out under aseptic conditions approaching those for surgery but in recent times there has been a tendency to use less stringent methods. The appearance of acquired immune deficiency syndrome (AIDS) and the potential for cross-infection with the human immuno-deficiency virus (HIV), formerly called the HTLVIII, from infected patients make it essential to re-examine the techniques used.

It is established that AIDS is associated with the HIV virus and that infection has occurred by transfer of the virus in blood or blood products. Much of the detail of the epidemiology and clinical pattern of the disease remain to be defined but enough is known to make sound recommendations for the precautions necessary. The majority of individuals both in America and Europe infected with HIV virus have been male homosexuals and it is established that receptive anal intercourse carries a major risk of infection. There are substantial numbers of haemophiliacs who have acquired the virus through receiving contaminated blood or blood products and an increasing number of intravenous drug addicts have become infected. HIV virus has also been isolated from most human bodily secretions including breast milk, tears, saliva and semen. There are grounds for believing that the virus is only intermittently present in most of these secretions but the blood of infected individuals is probably always infectious. The incubation period before the antibody becomes detectable in blood is about 42 days but it is not yet certain how variable this is, nor what proportion of antibody tests are falsely negative. It is too early to decide whether the risk of transfer of infection by tears or saliva is negligible. The HIV virus is of the retrovirus group and displays the appropriate properties, being labile and fragile. Outside its hosts it is easily destroyed by simple sterilization techniques. It is susceptible within 30 minutes to wet sterilization at 56°C, although a much longer period is required for dry sterilization. It is destroyed by strong hypochlorite solutions (domestic bleach) and by glutaraldehyde if instruments are immersed for 30 minutes. Most significantly, from the moment of infection with the virus the individual becomes infectious and remains so indefinitely. Screening procedures with testing for HIV virus antibody have been introduced in certain areas and hospitals, but they cannot provide complete protection of staff against the hazards of infection, as infected individuals who have not converted to HIV positive when antibody tested, or who give false negative results will continue to constitute an infectious risk. Prevention also relies upon medical or paramedical staff recognizing individuals who carry the infection from their social characteristics or previous treatment. Other major problems accompanying the introduction of screening procedures include any legal implications, and it is already established practice in the UK to refuse life insurance cover to individuals known to be HIV antibody positive.

The most logical policy to adopt for control of potential infection of staff is to introduce practices for universal use which avoid all possibility of infection from patients. It has been previous practice in both the US and UK to designate certain bronchoscopes or other instruments 'dirty' and restrict these for use where patients were known to be HIV antibody positive or suspected to be infected. While precautions adopted with such 'high risk patients' have been perfectly satisfactory it is illogical to adopt such adequate standards of cleanliness and hygiene and not use them universally for all patients. When such precautions are only used for recognized 'high risk patients', staff are still exposed to the dangers of infections from patients who are HIV-infected but thought not to be carriers because they have none of the obvious social stigmata. By using simple means for effective limitation of potential infection of staff and other patients the danger of unrecognized HIV virus carriers will be avoided. Until such time as it becomes clear that infection of staff by contamination with tears, saliva and other bodily secretions from patients with HIV virus is not a risk it should be assumed that these are hazardous. Such measures need not lead to the adoption of onerous changes in practice. The following methods are suggested for the use at all bronchoscopies:

1 The bronchoscopist and assistant should wear disposable or washable gowns, disposable gloves and eye protection in the form of close-fitting spectacles or goggles. The operator at least should wear a surgical mask to prevent contamination by droplet infection into the mouth.

2 All bronchoscopes, biopsy forceps and other instruments should be totally immersible and following routine cleansing should be sterilized by 30 minutes immersion in glutaraldehyde. It is clearly desirable to use the totally immersible newer generation instruments.

3 The previous use of ethylene oxide sterilization of bronchoscopes and biopsy forceps appears unnecessary now that the fragility and lability of the HIV virus is established.

4 All detritus including swabs from the bronchoscopy should be disposed of as though potentially infected.

5 All contaminated surfaces should be cleansed down with a 10% solution of household bleach.

6 Specimens obtained at bronchoscopy should be double bagged in heavy-duty polythene bags and carried to the laboratory upright.

7 The practice of biohazard labelling should be abandoned since this will not obviate risks from unrecognized infected individuals.

If subsequent studies show that the hazards of aerosol infection and transfer of non-blood containing secretions are negligible these policies can be reviewed. While it is recognized that at present HIV infection is relatively restricted to certain areas within the UK it is predicted that the world epidemic will continue as infection is likely to spread outside the present pool of male homosexuals, drug abusers and haemophiliacs.

Index